Biologic and Nanoarthroscopic Approaches in Sports Medicine

Chad Lavender
Editor

Biologic and Nanoarthroscopic Approaches in Sports Medicine

Springer

Editor
Chad Lavender
Orthopaedic Surgery Sports Medicine
Marshall University
Scott Depot, WV
USA

ISBN 978-3-030-71322-5 ISBN 978-3-030-71323-2 (eBook)
https://doi.org/10.1007/978-3-030-71323-2

This Springer imprint is published by the registered company Springer Nature Switzerland AG
The registered company address is: Gewerbestrasse 11, 6330 Cham, Switzerland

Foreword

It is an honor to write the foreword for Dr. Chad Lavender's first of what will likely be many books. It is thrilling and with great pride that we, the faculty members and past graduates of Orthopedic Research of Virginia, see and read this incredible book filled with state-of-the-art arthroscopic techniques. The highlights of the book are its educational insights into appropriate uses of orthobiologics and their application with the most minimally invasive tool to date, the nanoscope. While much research has been done and is yet to be done, the road map is clear, orthobiologics will continue to play a greater and greater role in the treatment of orthopedic pathologies. The procedure presentations starting with the ACL and then the nanoscope are stunning. Surely you will agree, Dr. Lavender and his talented host of contributors are deserving of our utmost congratulations on a job well done. It has been truly fascinating over the past 30 years to have witnessed the "age of the arthroscope." Many books and articles have chronicled the unprecedented march of technology and this book beautifully adds to the timeline of success. The unparalleled developments in arthroscopy is the product of conscientious and tireless efforts of many pioneers. All of us have been the beneficiaries of these efforts and we all have pioneers who mentored and assisted us in our journey with the arthroscope. At ORV, we were blessed with mentors like Dick Caspari, Rick Meyers, and Terry Whipple. But let's not forget our many partners including our industry and scientific colleagues who have equally helped pave the way to ever improved patient care. In the ORV tradition of technique development and refinement, Dr. Lavender has pushed the envelope to logical and exciting new heights. These achievements remind us that it was not so long ago when Dr. Caspari developed the arthroscopic trans-glenoid shoulder stabilization and Dr. Whipple began the arthroscopic treatment of wrist instability. These are exciting times to be an arthroscopist, and this progress has advanced the arthroscope past the treatment of "sports injuries" to the treatment of common and uncommon orthopedic problems. Cheers to Chad and his fellow authors and cheers to the past, present, and future of arthroscopic surgery.

William R. Beach, MD
Director of Orthopaedic Research of Virginia
Former AANA President
Richmond, Virginia

Preface

"Never skip a step"

Dr. Chad Lavender

Dear colleagues,

As orthopedic surgeons specializing in sports medicine, we have a unique opportunity to see the outcomes of our work in the field of play. This drives us to improve our practices in order to help patients have faster recoveries and return to play at higher levels. We work in a high-risk, high-reward field and one that is constantly changing. Obviously, you would not be reading this text if you were not interested in the development of novel techniques, the use of the latest biologics and minimally invasive procedures. The ideas behind this book started with a single conversation between myself and several Arthrex representatives, Aaron Ferguson, Shawn George, and Tyler Walker discussing how to improve ACL techniques with the use of biologics. Now, 3 years later, this book is a combination of not just those procedures but also methods that use cutting-edge technologies, such as the nanoscope. We at Marshall University are striving to continue to create innovative techniques,

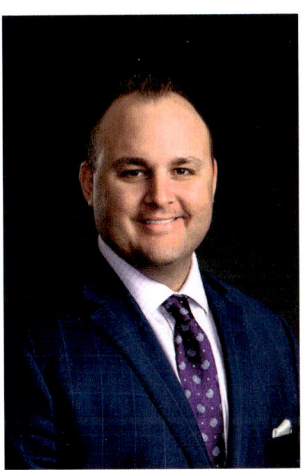

publish them, and help educate other surgeons on the utility and usefulness in order to incorporate them into practice.

Two parts create this book. Part one focuses on biologic advancement throughout different conditions. Part two focuses on nanoscopic techniques and how arthroscopy is changing into a more minimally invasive approach. Our hope is that surgeons will read this book and choose certain elements of the techniques in order to create new advancements to enhance our field. In this first edition, we are introducing new methods such as the use of biologics in ACL reconstruction, as well as introducing reconstructions and repairs using a nanoscope. We look forward to continuing to study the outcomes in clinical trials and refining the techniques as new technology arises.

I thank and acknowledge the patients and their families who have trusted us with their care while we develop these groundbreaking techniques. I also want to thank the residents, fellows, and attending physicians who have given their time to compose chapters for this book.

Scott Depot, WV, USA
Chad Lavender

Acknowledgements

I would like to take this opportunity to acknowledge all of those who have had a role in my training and my development as an orthopedic surgeon. I was fortunate to have remarkable coaches and professors at West Virginia University throughout undergraduate and medical school. Later, I began my residency at Marshall University, which provided me the opportunity to excel and train in orthopedics. Special thank you to Dr. Charles Giangarra, my biggest mentor. Additionally, I had an outstanding fellowship program at the Orthopaedic Research of Virginia. During fellowship, I developed the drive to create new techniques, which you will read in the following chapters. Certainly, without the authors of the chapters, I would be unable to present this book. Therefore, we are grateful for those at Marshall University, the residents, and attending physicians who have participated in composing this text. Also special thanks to Dr. Akhavan and his fellows at the Orthopaedic Sports Medicine Fellowship at Allegheny General Hospital as well as Dr. Caldwell and his fellows at the Orthopaedic Research of Virginia. I am very thankful that these two exceptional programs helped to facilitate the creation of the first edition of this book.

As it relates to the contents of this book and the creation of the techniques, numerous people have contributed in providing important tools and ideas, which helped refine these techniques. Special acknowledgments to our local representatives, Aaron Ferguson, Cameron Guill, and Mike Molina, as well as our regional representatives, Dave Hawkins, Shawn George, Tyler Walker, John Parulski, and Bart Kayser. I would also like to acknowledge the corporate representatives at Arthrex: Chelsea Day, Robert Benedict, Ryan Keller, and the owner Reinhold Schmieding. Each of these individuals played a role either in the day-to-day development of these techniques or the overall conceptualization of the techniques. They truly helped fuel our passion to enhance these methods, which ultimately will lead to improved patient outcomes.

It is especially important to acknowledge our sports team, both in the operating room and clinically. The OR staff has had patience as we developed each technique and continually revised them. It has not been easy to develop novel techniques and I can attest that each of them helped develop certain pearls that led to the success. I would also like to thank my staff in the clinic, starting with my nurse practitioner, Kara Cipriani, who has helped me with every aspect of our practice, including research for the past 6 years. Special thank you to Ginger Peters, my office manager who has worked tirelessly to maintain our high practice standards. Additionally, thank you to my other clinic staff who are involved in our daily activities. Many thanks to Chad Fisher and Dr. Ali Oliashirazi for their exceptional support and guidance in our clinical practice.

I would like to acknowledge my parents, David and Patty Lavender, who provided the opportunity for me to attend medical school to begin this journey and helped instill in me the characteristics that I still use today in practice. To my wife, Michelle, my son, Chance, and daughter, Louren, who have allowed me to spend thousands of hours on the videos and development of techniques, I am forever grateful. They truly have an understanding for my passion to improve patient outcomes.

Finally, and most importantly, I would like to acknowledge each of my athletes and patients who trusted me to perform and utilize the new techniques to enhance their recovery. They are an inspiration and make my career rewarding; it is because of them that I am able to provide you with this textbook.

Contents

Contributors

Syed Ali Sina Adil, MD PGY3 Marshall University, Scott Depot, WV, USA

Sam Akhavan, MD Orthopaedic Sports Medicine, Allegheny Health Network, Pittsburgh, PA, USA

Galen Berdis, MD PGY4 Marshall University, Scott Depot, WV, USA

Baylor Blickenstaff, MD Department of Orthopaedic Surgery, Marshall University, Scott Depot, WV, USA

Matthew Bullock, DO, MPT Department of Orthopaedic Surgery, Marshall University, Huntington, WV, USA

Paul E. Caldwell Orthopaedic Research of Virginia and Tuckahoe Orthopaedic Associates, Ltd., Richmond, VA, USA

Jeeshan A. Faridi, MD Orthopaedic Research of Virginia Sports Medicine Fellowship Program, Richmond, VA, USA

Kassandra Flores MS1 Marshall University, Scott Depot, WV, USA

Andrew Fontaine, MD PGY4 Marshall University, Huntington, WV, USA

William Scott Fravel, MD Department of Orthopaedic Surgery, Marshall University, Scott Depot, WV, USA

Charles Giangarra, MD Department of Orthopaedic Surgery, VA Medical Center, Marshall University School of Medicine, Huntington, WV, USA

John Jasko, MD Marshall University, Orthopaedic Surgery Sports Medicine, Huntington, WV, USA

Chad Lavender, MD Orthopaedic Surgery Sports Medicine, Marshall University, Scott Depot, WV, USA

Dana Lycans, MD Sports Medicine Division, Department of Orthopaedic Surgery, Marshall University School of Medicine, Huntington, West Virginia, USA

Sohaib Malik, MD Orthopedic Surgery Resident, Marshall University, Huntington, WV, USA

Ali Oliashirazi, MD Marshall University, Scott Depot, WV, USA

Tyag K. Patel, MD PGY3 Marshall University, Scott Depot, WV, USA

Vishavpreet Singh, MD PGY4 Marshall University, Scott Depot, WV, USA

Shane Taylor, MD PGY1 Marshall University, Scott Depot, WV, USA

Christopher Wang, MD Allegheny Health Network, Pittsburgh, PA, USA

Andrew Wilhelm, DO, DPT Orthopaedic Sports Medicine, Allegheny Health Network, Pittsburgh, PA, USA

Part I

Advanced Biologic Techniques in Sports Medicine

Biologics in Sports Medicine

Galen Berdis and John Jasko

1 Introduction

Over the past several years, the use of biologic therapies has become popular for a wide range of sports medicine injuries and other orthopedic-related diseases including tendon injury or inflammation, ligamentous injury, cartilaginous injury, and osteoarthritis. These biologic treatment options are often autologous in nature, of which the two most popular are platelet-rich plasma and mesenchymal stem cells that are most commonly harvested from bone marrow concentrate. The FDA does not currently regulate the use of bone marrow concentrate or platelet-rich plasma as they fall outside of the scope of what the FDA considers human cells, tissue, and cellular and tissue-based products (HCT/Ps) in title 21, part 1271, of the Code of Federal Regulations (CFR), and therefore the use of both PRP and BMC has been expanding in clinical practice [1]. It is important that both PRP and BMC should be registered and taken through the proper protocols established by the FDA [2, 3].

2 Platelet-Rich Plasma

PRP is made up of platelets, plasma, leukocytes, monocytes, and neutrophils each with associated growth factors [4]. As the most numerous cell in PRP, platelets release substantial amounts of insulin-like growth factor 1 (IGF-1), transforming growth factor β (TGF-β), platelet-derived growth factor (PDGF), fibroblast growth factor (FGF), epidermal growth factor (EGF), and vascular endothelial growth

G. Berdis (✉)
Marshall University, Huntington, WV, USA

J. Jasko
Marshall University, Orthopaedic Surgery Sports Medicine, Huntington, WV, USA
e-mail: jasko@marshall.edu

C. Lavender (ed.), *Biologic and Nanoarthroscopic Approaches in Sports Medicine*, https://doi.org/10.1007/978-3-030-71323-2_1

factor (VEGF) [4]. The rationale behind the use of PRP for treatment is that platelets are the first to arrive at the site of tissue injury and thus have the potential to release growth factors that play a critical role in mediating healing [5]. PRP has been used during surgery at sites of tendon repair and reconstructions such as rotator cuff repairs and anterior cruciate ligament (ACL) reconstructions.

3 Bone Marrow Concentrate

Bone marrow concentrate (BMC) differs from PRP in that it attempts to harness the healing value of mesenchymal stem cells. Bone marrow has become an excellent source to harvest stem cells due to its easy accessibility and sufficient quantities for clinical use without the need for ex vivo expansion [6]. For clinical use, bone marrow may be harvested as can be read in several techniques throughout this book, and concentrated through a method involving centrifugation. Through the development of the Arthrex (Naples, Fl) Angel system BMC can now be harvested and used during surgery within minutes. There are several sites to harvest bone marrow, but we prefer the proximal tibia for knee procedures. A second major source of MSCs which is used in clinical practice is adipose tissue, which is not discussed in this chapter as it is not a current source of MSCs in the techniques described in later chapters [7]. The rationale behind the use of BMC derived MSCs is that these cells have the potential to regenerate tissue directly through differentiation into cell lineages of the tissues in which they are placed such as damaged ligament, tendon or cartilage and may indirectly facilitate healing through stimulation of angiogenesis and recruiting local tissue-specific progenitors [8].

4 Clinical Use of PRP and BMC

Despite inconsistent evidence to support the use of PRP and BMC for the treatment of various sports-related injuries, their clinical use has been wide and continues to expand. Current indications include use during ligament reconstruction to promote healing response, promotion of healing response in tendinopathy, use in treatment of osteoarthritis, and treatment of osteochondral damage.

The use of biologics in ACL reconstruction has been studied but mainly centered on the use of PRP. A systematic review conducted by Vavken et al. which included eight studies found that "the addition of platelet concentrates to ACL reconstruction may have a beneficial effect on graft maturation and could improve it by 20–30% on average" [9]. In an MRI-based single-blinded prospective study, regarding time to tendon healing, Radice et al. found that PRP augmented ACL reconstruction required only 48% of the time to achieve a homogenous healed graft compared to non-PRP group [10]. Vascular endothelial growth factor (VEGF), which can be found in PRP, has been studied in its role for angiogenesis in ACL reconstruction. Takayama et al. demonstrated that blocking VEGF will reduce angiogenesis after ACL reconstruction, prevent graft maturation, and reduce biomechanical strength following ACL reconstruction [11]. Throughout this book you will see BMC used in a variety of applications to hopefully improve ligament and cartilage reconstructions and repairs. The theory is BMC will show even enhanced results from those focused on PRP and VEGF mentioned above.

PRP and BMC have been used in clinical practice to treat tendon injury and tendinopathy although there is limited evidence of improved outcomes in the literature. In a recent meta-analysis of the use of biologics in rotator cuff pathology, Randelli et al. concluded that 13 clinical trials from 2011 to 2014 utilizing PRP for rotator cuff tear repairs have provided controversial results and that research regarding the use of MSCs in shoulder surgery is limited [12]. The single identified human pilot trial in the meta-analysis was performed by Ellera Gomes et al. which enrolled 14 patients who underwent augmented RTC repair with autologous bone marrow concentrate aspirated from iliac crest with all 14 patients showing tendon integrity at minimum 12-month follow up on MRI [13].

Epicondylitis has been a common application of the use of PRP, with lateral epicondylitis more extensively studied than medial. A meta-analysis was performed by Arirachakaran et al. in 2016 which identified ten studies that met inclusion criteria. The authors concluded that PRP significantly improved pain and Patient-Related Tennis Elbow Evaluation scores when compared with autologous blood or corticosteroid injection for the treatment of lateral epicondylitis [14]. BMC has been less extensively studied for use in tendinopathy than PRP; however, one small study with 8 patients at 5-year follow up showed that 7 out of 8 patients had excellent results after ultrasound-guided inoculation of the patellar tendon from iliac crest harvested bone marrow concentrate [15].

Many practitioners have begun to utilize PRP and BMC in their treatment of knee osteoarthritis. In their literature review, Lamplot et al. identified 12 level 1 studies that utilized platelet-rich plasma in the setting of knee osteoarthritis many of which show promising results for pain and knee scores when comparing PRP to hyaluronic acid or saline placebo control [16]. A systematic review by Chalha et al. identified 11 studies of BMC use in knee OA and osteochondral injuries. Three of these studies showed good or excellent results for BMC use in knee OA and 8 of the studies showed good or excellent results in the treatment of focal chondral defects [17]. At this time, the American Academy of Orthopaedic Surgeons (AAOS) in their clinical practice guidelines currently does not recommend for or against the use of PRP for the treatment of knee osteoarthritis due to lack of sufficient evidence.

Despite the lack of conclusive evidence regarding the benefit of PRP and BMC use in the aforementioned sports-related pathology, there have been very promising results in the literature that warrant further well-designed randomized controlled trials. Surgeons continue to treat patients with PRP and BMC and have developed new and exciting surgical techniques to utilize their healing potential. This book demonstrates many different emerging techniques for the treatment of sports-related injuries and will highlight the use of biologics with various surgical interventions.

References

1. Food and Drug Administration. Regulatory Considerations for Human Cells, Tissues and Cellular and Tissue-Based Products: Minimal Manipulation and Homologous Use. Washington, DC: US Department of Health and Human Services; 2017.
2. LaPrade RF, Geeslin AG, Murray IR, et al. Biologic treatments for sports injuries II think tank – Current concepts, future research, and barriers to advancement, part 1: Biologics overview, ligament injury, tendinopathy. Am. J. Sports Med. 2016;44(12):3270–83.
3. Food and Drug Administration. Guidance for Industry Current Good Tissue Practice (CGTP) and Additional Requirements for Manufacturers of Human Cells, Tissues, and Cellular and Tissue-Based Products (HCT/Ps). Washington, DC: US Department of Health and Human Services; 2011.
4. Wasterlain AS, Braun HJ, Dragoo JL. Contents and formulations of platelet-rich plasma. Operat Tech Orthop. 2012;22:33–42.
5. Creaney L, HamiltonGrowth B. Factor delivery methods in the management of sports injuries: The state of play. Br. J. Sports Med. 2008;42:314–20.
6. Murray IR, Corselli M, Petrigliano FA, Soo C, Peault B. Recent insights into the identity of mesenchymal stem cells: Implications for orthopaedic applications. Bone Joint J. 2014;96(3):291–8.
7. Aust L, Devlin B, Foster SJ. Yield of human adipose-derived adult stem cells from liposuction aspirates. Cytotherapy. 2004;6(1):7–14.
8. Anz AW, Hackel JG, Nilssen EC, Andrews JR. Application of biologics in the treatment of the rotator cuff, meniscus, cartilage, and osteoarthritis. J. Am. Acad. Orthop. Surg. 2014;22(2):68–79.
9. Vavken P, Sadoghi P, Murray MM. The effect of platelet concentrates on graft maturation and graft-bone interface healing in anterior cruciate ligament reconstruction in human patients: A systematic review of controlled trials. Arthroscopy. 2011;27(11):1573–83.
10. Radice F, Yanez R, Gutierrez V, Rosales J, Pinedo M, Coda S. Comparison of magnetic resonance imaging findings in anterior cruciate ligament grafts with and without autologous platelet-derived growth factors. Arthroscopy. 2010;26(1):50–7.
11. Takayama K, Kawakami Y, Mifune Y, et al. The effect of blocking angiogenesis on anterior cruciate ligament healing following stem cell transplantation. Biomaterials. 2015;60:9–19.
12. Randelli P, Randelli F, Ragone V, et al. Regenerative medicine in rotator cuff injuries. Biomed. Res. Int. 2014;2014:129515.
13. Ellera Gomes JL, da Silva RC, Silla LM, Abreu MR, Pellanda R. Conventional rotator cuff repair complemented by the aid of mononuclear autologous stem cells. Knee Surg. Sports Traumatol. Arthrosc. 2012;20(2):373–7.
14. Arirachakaran A, Sukthuayat A, Sisayanarane T, Laoratanavoraphong S, Kanchanatawan W, Kongtharvonskul J. Platelet-rich plasma versus autologous blood versus steroid injection in lateral epicondylitis: Systematic review and network meta-analysis. J. Orthop. Traumatol. 2016;17(2):101–12.
15. Pascual-Garrido C, Rolon A, Makino A. Treatment of chronic patellar tendinopathy with autologous bone marrow stem cells: A 5-year follow up. Stem Cells Int. 2012;2012:953510.
16. Lamplot JD, Rodeo SA, Brophy RH. A practical guide for the current use of biologic therapies in sports medicine. Am. J. Sports Med. 2020 Feb;48(2):488–503.
17. Chahla J, Dean CS, Moatshe G, Pascual-Garrido C, Serra Cruz R, LaPrade RF. Concentrated bone marrow aspirate for the treatment of chondral injuries and osteoarthritis of the knee: A systematic review of outcomes. Orthop. J. Sports Med. 2016;4(1):2325967115625481.

Augmentation of Bone Patella Tendon Bone ACL Reconstruction with BMC and a Suture Tape and the Rationale Behind Biologic ACL Reconstructions

Vishavpreet Singh and Chad Lavender

1 Introduction

Graft rerupture is one of the major complications and causes of reoperation after anterior cruciate ligament (ACL) reconstruction. This is more common in younger athletes. On the basis of the recent literature, the rate of graft rerupture is about 6–11% [1]. Even with newer techniques and different types of grafts, the rerupture rates and return-to-play period have not been improved significantly. Athletes younger than 25 years old have been found to have a 23% risk of secondary ACL injury on either the contralateral or ipsilateral side after an ACL reconstruction [2]. Therefore, there is a direct need to improve the outcomes of ACL reconstruction especially in younger athletes. This could be accomplished with earlier biologic incorporation of the graft and further protection of the graft during the early postoperative period. Bone-patellar tendon-bone (BPTB) autograft reconstruction is widely considered the gold standard for younger athletes receiving surgery. Recently, autogenous bone marrow aspirate was shown to have superior radiographic incorporation when used for osteochondral allograft transplantation in the knee [3]. Bone marrow aspirate was also shown to have similar mesenchymal stem cell concentrations when harvested from the proximal tibia compared with when

With permission from Arthroscopy Techniques, Lavender C, Johnson B, Kopiec A. Augmentation of anterior cruciate ligament with bone marrow concentrate and a suture tape. *Arthrosc Tech* 2018;7:e1289–1293.

V. Singh
PGY4 Marshall University, Scott Depot, WV, USA
e-mail: singhv@marshall.edu

C. Lavender (✉)
Orthopaedic Surgery Sports Medicine, Marshall University, Scott Depot, WV, USA

C. Lavender (ed.), *Biologic and Nanoarthroscopic Approaches in Sports Medicine*, https://doi.org/10.1007/978-3-030-71323-2_2

harvested from the iliac crest, providing a useful and safe alternative during knee surgery [4]. This bone marrow concentrate can be combined with demineralized bone matrix as a medium for incorporation into a femoral tunnel during ACL reconstruction. In addition, suture tape augmentation (Arthrex, Naples, FL) was recently used for ACL allograft reconstruction and found to be safe and effective [5]. This chapter describes our technique for augmentation of BPTB autograft ACL reconstruction with bone marrow concentrate mixed with Allosync Pure (Arthrex), as well as the addition of suture tape augmentation (Arthrex) for early strength.

2 Indications

The indications for biologic and suture tape augmentation of an ACL reconstruction include patients at increased risk of rerupture. This patient population comprises young active athletes playing competitive sports, as well as patients undergoing revision ACL reconstruction. We also think this technique is indicated in patients attempting to return to play more quickly than 7–9 months after surgery.

3 Contraindications

Our technique is contraindicated in patients with open physes, as well as patients with severe tunnel enlargement from previous surgery in need of bone grafting.

4 Surgical Technique

4.1 Patient Setup

The patient is placed supine in a standard knee arthroscopy position. The operative extremity is placed into a leg holder with a tourniquet applied to the thigh, and the nonoperative extremity is placed on a well-leg pillow.

4.2 Bone Marrow Aspiration

Before inflation of the tourniquet, a small stab incision is made just lateral to the tibial tubercle. An aspiration needle and central sharp trocar are inserted while angled 10 proximally (Fig. 1). A mark is made on the needle at 30 mm to avoid over insertion. The central trocar is removed, and the first few milliliters of aspirate is discarded because of the excess amount of bone. Then, 60 mL of bone marrow is aspirated into heparinized syringes (Fig. 2).

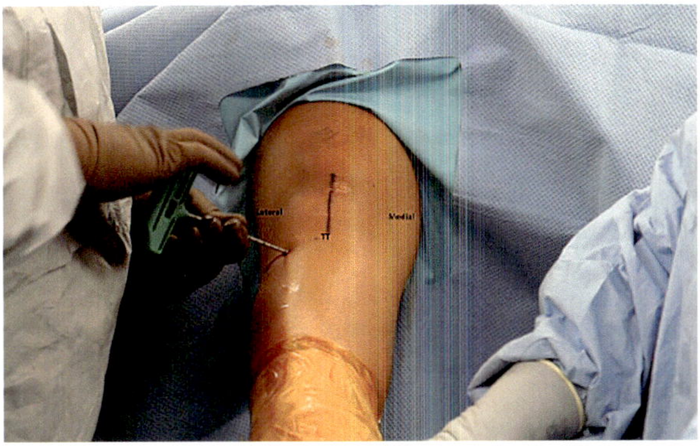

Fig. 1 The patient's right knee is placed supine, and the aspiration needle with the trocar is inserted slightly lateral to the tibial tubercle angled 10° proximally. Insertion past a depth of 30 mm should not occur

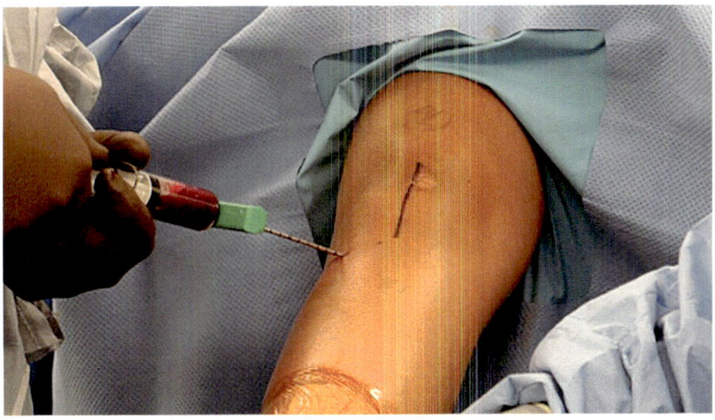

Fig. 2 While the patient is still supine, after insertion of the aspiration needle, the central trocar is removed. Then, 60 mL of bone marrow is aspirated into heparinized syringes

4.3 Mixing Bone Marrow Aspirate with Allosync Pure

After aspiration of the bone marrow, the aspirate is concentrated using the Arthrex Angel device, and a total of 3 mL of bone marrow is mixed by hand with 5 mL of Allosync Pure. This mixture is then placed into an arthroscopic cannula delivery device.

4.4 ACL Technique

The tourniquet is inflated, and a standard diagnostic arthroscopy reveals the ACL rupture. A standard BPTB graft harvest is performed to achieve a graft length of 89 mm with 20-mm bone blocks. Two No. 2 FiberWire sutures (Arthrex) are placed tangentially to each other in the tibial bone block, while the BTB TightRope button system (Arthrex) is placed into the femoral-sided bone block. The TightRope system should be loosened to add more length so that the surgeon can later flip the button on the femur and still have space available to inject the bone marrow graft into the femur before bringing the graft into the joint. At this point, after loosening the system, we place the suture tape augmentation (InternalBrace; Arthrex) through the button opposite the passing suture in the TightRope (Fig. 3). The remnants of the ACL are debrided, and the FlipCutter (Arthrex) is used to make a femoral socket length of 30 mm in the standard location. After the femoral socket is made, a No. 2 FiberStick (Arthrex) is passed into the joint and docked outside the lateral portal until the tibial tunnel is completed. The tibial tunnel is also created with the FlipCutter, and it may be helpful to open the anterior surface of the tibia with an opening reamer. The passing suture is brought out of the tibial tunnel. By use of the passing suture, the femoral TightRope portion is brought into the joint and then flipped on the lateral cortex of the femur.

4.5 Bone Marrow Graft Passage

Before the ACL graft is brought into the joint, the InternalBrace is retrieved and docked outside the medial portal (Fig. 4). The arthroscopic cannula is placed through the medial portal, and the knee is hyperflexed. The graft is injected into the femoral tunnel to fill approximately half of the tunnel (Figs. 5 and 6). The ACL graft

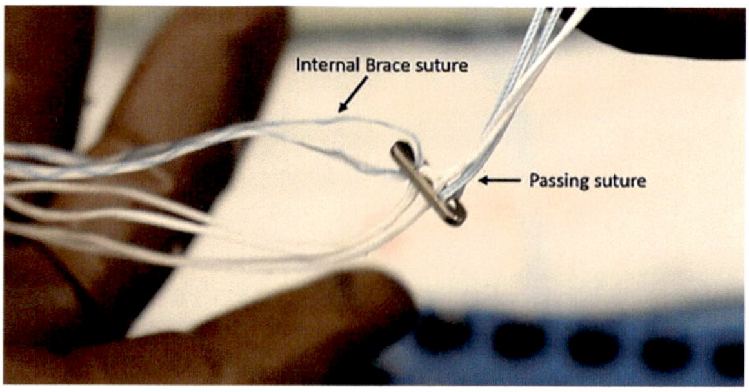

Fig. 3 The TightRope system has been loosened to allow more length between the graft and button. The InternalBrace is threaded through the hole in the TightRope button opposite the blue passing sutures. It may be helpful to use a passing wire or needle

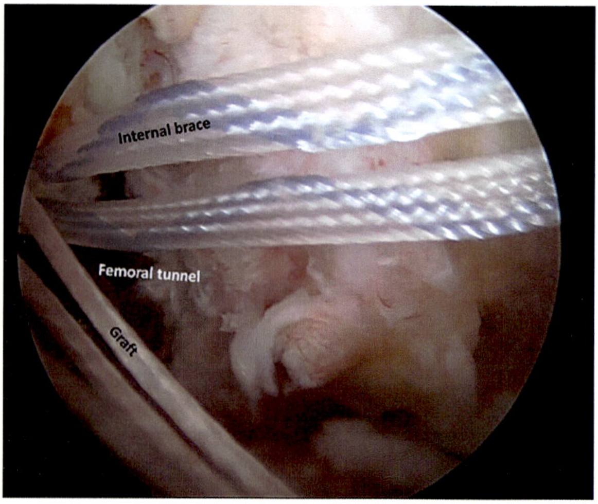

Fig. 4 Viewing with the 30° arthroscope from the anterolateral portal, the InternalBrace has been retrieved from the medial portal before the graft is passed into the joint and before the bone marrow graft is injected into the tunnel

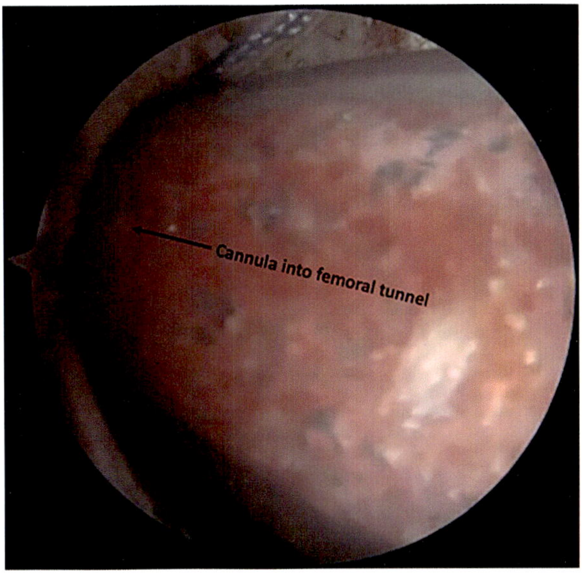

Fig. 5 The patient's right knee is flexed to 90° and may need to be hyperflexed. Viewing from the anterolateral portal, the arthroscopic cannula is used to injection bone marrow graft into the femoral tunnel

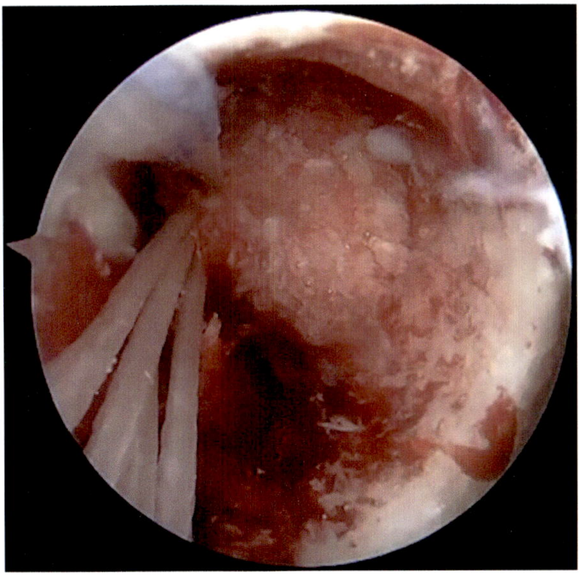

Fig. 6 Viewing the right knee with the 30° arthroscope from the anteromedial portal, looking into the femoral tunnel, half of the tunnel has been filled with the bone marrow graft

is pulled into the femoral tunnel using alternating pulls on the white sutures coming out of the TightRope device (Fig. 7). The ACL graft is then fixed at 30° of extension in standard fashion on the tibia with a 9 × 23 mm BioComposite interference screw (Arthrex). The screw should be as anterior as possible to help locate the wire within the joint.

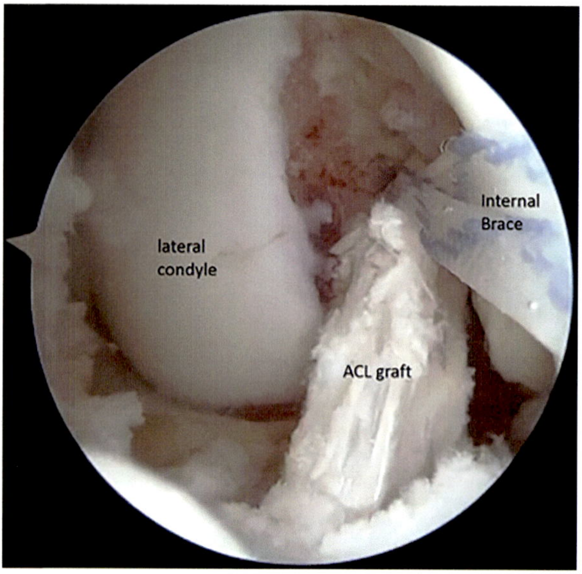

Fig. 7 Viewing the right knee in 90° of flexion with the 30° arthroscope from the anteromedial portal, the anterior cruciate ligament (ACL) graft has been pulled from the tibial tunnel and tensioned into the femoral tunnel in standard fashion. It should be noted that no bone marrow graft was displaced into the knee joint

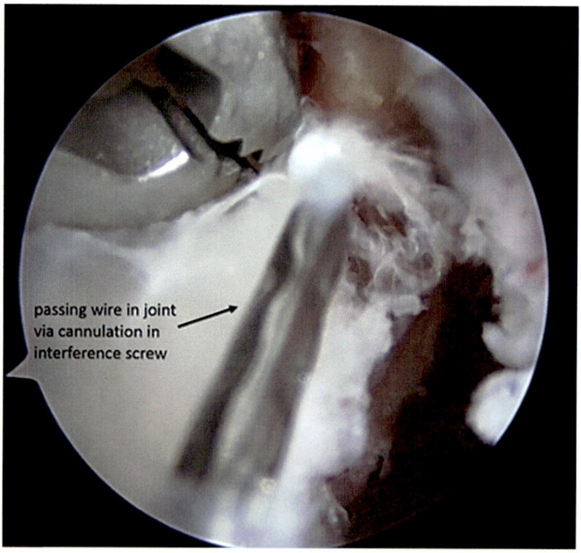

Fig. 8 Viewing the right knee with the 30° arthroscope from the anteromedial portal, the passing wire is located within the joint and retrieved through the medial portal with the InternalBrace, which had been docked in that portal

4.6 InternalBrace Passage and Fixation

After placing the interference screw, the surgeon leaves the driver in the screw and passes a wire with a loop through the cannulation. This wire is then located within the joint (Fig. 8). The wire is retrieved through the medial portal along with the

InternalBrace, and the InternalBrace is threaded through the loop in the wire. The wire is then pulled through the tibial screw, and the InternalBrace follows the wire (Fig. 9). The InternalBrace and tibial bone block sutures are threaded through a 4.75-mm SwiveLock anchor (Arthrex), and the SwiveLock is fixed on the anterior surface of the tibia in standard fashion at 0° of extension (Fig. 10). Table 1 lists advantages and disadvantages of our technique, and Table 2 presents technical pearls.

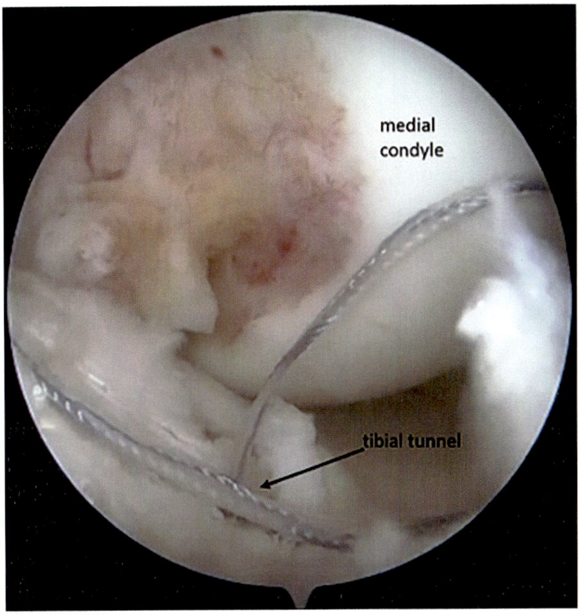

Fig. 9 Viewing the right knee in 90° of flexion with the 30° arthroscope from the anterolateral portal, the InternalBrace is passed using the passing wire through the tibial interference screw

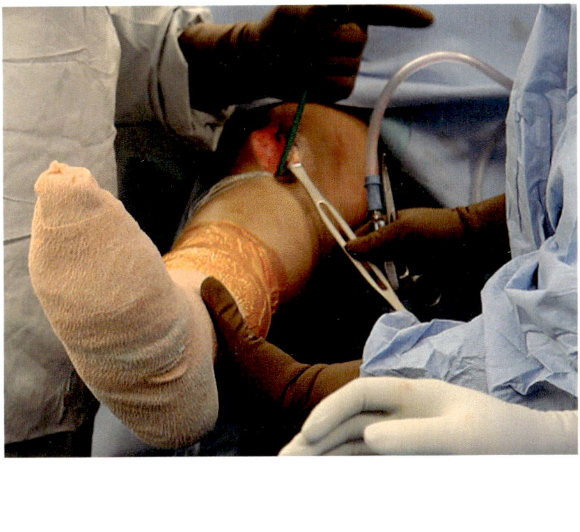

Fig. 10 With the right knee supine and the knee in 30° of flexion, the InternalBrace is placed through a SwiveLock anchor and the anchor is fixed in standard fashion on the anteromedial surface of the tibia

Table 1 Advantages and disadvantages of bone marrow concentrate and suture tape augmentation in ACL reconstruction

Advantages
Bone marrow harvesting can be performed at a site that has already been prepared and draped
Stem cells and bone grafting may lead to stronger and more substantial graft incorporation in the femoral tunnel
Remaining bone graft can be used to fill the defects in the patella and tibia from graft harvest, which may decrease anterior knee pain
Suture tape augmentation could lead to improved early outcomes and possibly an earlier return to play for athletes
Disadvantages
Increased cost
Increased operating room time
Added incision from bone marrow harvest site
Increased risk of fracture due to addition of aspiration site to tibia

Table 2 Technical pearls of bone marrow concentrate and suture tape augmentation in ACL reconstruction

Aspirate the bone marrow before the tourniquet is inflated
If the syringe stops filling during bone marrow aspiration, rotate the aspiration needle
Place the interference screw anterior to help with locating the passing wire
Use a cannula to prevent a suture bridge when passing the InternalBrace. Use suture tape (InternalBrace) rather than FiberTape (Arthrex)

5 Rehabilitation

We use our standard ACL rehabilitation protocol. The patient is placed in a hinged knee brace locked in full extension until full quadriceps control is achieved. The patient is allowed full weight bearing in the brace immediately after surgery. In our protocol, early passive range of motion with formal physical therapy is started within the first week. The patient is then progressed through strengthening with standard ACL rehabilitation techniques.

6 Discussion

BPTB autograft ACL reconstruction is widely accepted as the gold standard in treating young athletes with ACL ruptures. Rerupture and return to play are still concerning issues facing younger high-risk patients. Currently, there are very few techniques involving biologic augmentation of the ACL reconstruction. The advantages of the described technique include the location of harvesting through a site that has already been prepared and draped. This adds very little surgical time to the operation, and the graft can be injected arthroscopically. The stem cells and bone grafting should lead to stronger and more substantial graft incorporation in the femoral tunnel. The remaining graft can also be used to fill the defects in the patella and tibia from graft harvest and may lead to less pain. If we consider a socket to be a pot and the ACL graft to be a plant, then the addition of mesenchymal stem cells as we have described should be termed a "fertilized" ACL. There are some added risks with this procedure primarily from the addition of the bone marrow aspiration site. This additional harvest site could be a source of postoperative pain. Theoretically, there is an added risk of fracture because of the addition of the aspiration site to the tibia, although we believe this is a limited risk. One limitation of this technique is the cost it adds to the operation; however, we believe the benefits are worth the cost in young patients at high risk of rerupture and in revision cases. Another limitation is the increased difficulty the technique adds to the standard ACL reconstruction. Although our technique has risks and limitations, we believe this will improve patient outcomes especially in those at risk of complications. When the biologic advantages of the bone marrow graft are combined with the strength of the suture tape augmentation, we believe this could lead to improved early outcomes and possibly an earlier return to play for these athletes. In these high-risk populations, this is now our procedure of choice for ACL reconstruction [6].

7 Editor's View

Throughout this book you will see an evolution of different techniques and a variety of biologics and minimally invasive surgical techniques. This technique in particular was the first of our series of biologic techniques involving ACL reconstruction. It was very important for us to start with a gold standard BTB technique and utilize biologics into the reconstruction and you can see that we fertilized the femoral tunnel with BMC and Allosync Pure and also important about this technique is how we pass the internal brace through the actual interference crew. I have not found an issue with placing too much of the biologic mixture to create a graft mismatch issue. It is important to remember that the bone block is more dense than the composite graft. We feel that this is a great option for those that want the BTB but also would like to utilize biologics in their reconstructions. In a very active athlete who you would like to use a BTB graft because it is considered the gold standard I think this is a great option and a way to stay up to date with the current biologic techniques.

References

1. Crawford SN, Waterman BR, Lubowitz JH. Long-term failure of anterior cruciate ligament reconstruction. Arthroscopy. 2013;39:1566–71.
2. Wiggins AJ, Grandhi RK, Schneider DK, Stanfield D, Webster KE, Myer GD. Risk of secondary injury in younger athletes after anterior cruciate ligament reconstruction: a systematic review and meta-analysis. Am J Sports Med. 2016;44:1861–76.
3. Oladeji LO, Stannard JP, Cook CR, et al. Effects of autogenous bone marrow aspirate concentrate on radiographic integration of femoral condylar osteochondral allografts. Am J Sports Med. 2017;45:2793–803.

4. Narbona-Carceles J, Vaquero J, Suárez-Sancho S, Forriol F, Fernández-Santos ME. Bone marrow mesenchymal stem cell aspirates from alternative sources: is the knee as good as the iliac crest? Injury. 2014;45:S42–7.
5. Smith PA, Bley JA. Allograft anterior cruciate ligament reconstruction utilizing internal brace augmentation. Arthrosc Tech. 2016;5:e1143–7.
6. Lavender C, Johnson B, Kopiec A. Augmentation of anterior cruciate ligament with bone marrow concentrate and a suture tape. Arthrosc Tech. 2018;7:e1289–93.

All-Inside Allograft ACL Reconstruction Augmented with Amnion, BMC, and a Suture Tape

Tyag K. Patel, Dana Lycans, and Chad Lavender

1 Introduction

Among young athletes, anterior cruciate ligament (ACL) rupture is one of the most common ligamentous knee injuries, particularly in those sports requiring cutting and jumping movements [1–5]. It is estimated that over 100,000 athletes annually will require reconstructive surgery to avoid chronic instability and chondral injury [1–5]. Graft re-rupture is a major complication affecting many of these athletes, with estimated rates of 6–11% [6]. Despite changes in surgical technique and graft choice, these rates have not changed significantly over time [7]. The current hope is that by developing techniques that hasten biologic incorporation, re-rupture rates and functional outcomes can be improved.

Due to advances in tissue engineering, biologic augmentation of the graft with amnion may further improve graft incorporation [8, 9]. Although amniotic membrane-derived products have yet to be studied in ligament reconstruction of the knee, they have been shown to be effective in the realms of plastic surgery and ophthalmology, providing a theoretical basis for use [10].

With permission from Arthroscopy Techniques: Lavender C, Bishop C. The Fertilized Anterior Cruciate Ligament: An All-Inside Anterior Cruciate Ligament Reconstruction Augmented with Amnion, Bone Marrow Concentrate, and a Suture Tape. *Arthroscopic Techniques* 2019; 8: e555–e559.

T. K. Patel
PGY3 Marshall University, Scott Depot, WV, USA
e-mail: patelt@marshall.edu

D. Lycans
Sports Medicine Division, Department of Orthopaedic Surgery, Marshall University School of Medicine, Huntington, West Virginia, USA
e-mail: lycans@marshall.edu

C. Lavender (✉)
Orthopaedic Surgery Sports Medicine, Marshall University, Scott Depot, WV, USA

C. Lavender (ed.), *Biologic and Nanoarthroscopic Approaches in Sports Medicine*, https://doi.org/10.1007/978-3-030-71323-2_3

In addition, a recent study reported that when used with osteochondral allografts, bone marrow concentrate showed superior radiographic outcomes in the knee [11]. By combining this concentrate with Allosync Pure (Arthrex, Naples, FL) to graft both the femoral and tibial tunnels, the goal is to improve graft incorporation. We call this grafting of the tunnels fertilizing the acl. If you think of the acl like a plant you are placing in a pot (socket) then we are adding fertilizer to this construct. In this chapter, we continue on the idea of the previous chapter in which we fertilized the femoral tunnel of a btb acl reconstruction.

By using bone marrow concentrate and amnion together with the use of a suture tape (Arthrex, Naples, FL), the belief is that failure rates and functional outcomes can be improved [12]. In addition, there are early advantages to an all-inside ACL reconstruction such as decreased pain, and when this is combined with biologics, we may be able to accelerate rehabilitation and return to play more than previously anticipated. This chapter describes a complete biologic ACL reconstruction designed to enhance graft bone integration, in addition to faster and improved vascularization of the graft.

2 Indications

Currently, we use this technique in high demand and active patients over the age of 25 when allograft is used. You can use amnion as well with quad tendon grafts or other all inside techniques. Any case you would like to use all biologics available such as revision settings this technique is a great option.

3 Contraindications

Allograft is not currently recommended in those young athletes at high risk of re-rupture, but you could still use the amnion and fertilization process in those patients with a quadriceps or hamstring graft link construct.

4 Technique

4.1 Amnion and Graft Preparation

A standard graft-link allograft is prepared, and the femoral-sided suspensory fixation loop is lengthened to allow space for injection of the composite graft into the femoral tunnel later in the case. With the epithelial side facing up, the 3 × 6 mm amnion is wrapped around the central portion of the graft (Fig. 1). By use of No. 4-0 Vicryl (Ethicon, Somerville, NJ), a standard loop stitch is placed 1 mm from each end of the amnion and tied. These stitches will help seal the amnion. With the use of the same No. 4-0 Vicryl suture, a baseball stitch is then placed in the seam created where the amnion edge is to complete the seal (Fig. 2).

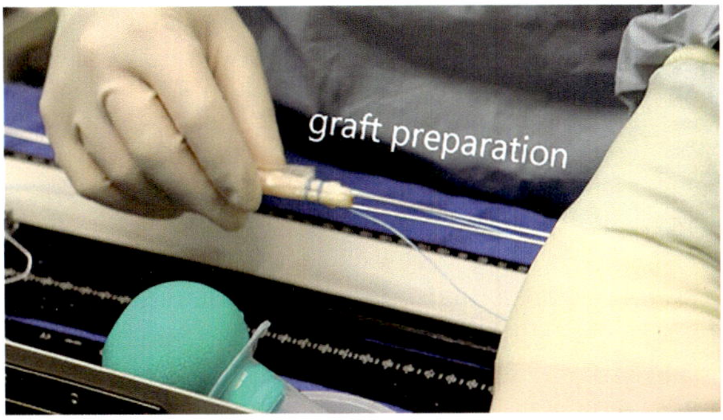

Fig. 1 Standard graft-link allograft while wrapping amnion circumferentially around graft

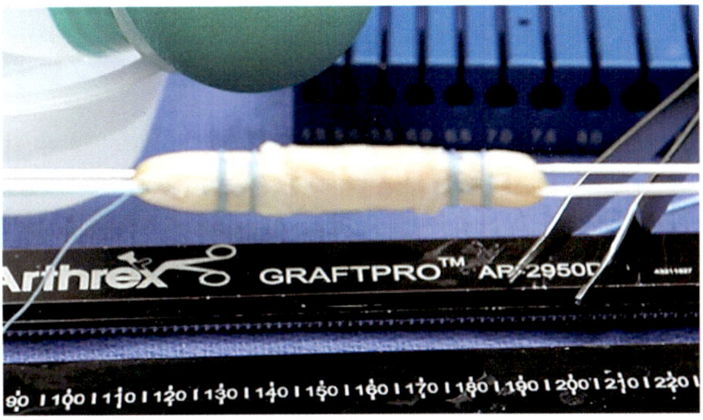

Fig. 2 Graft on preparation station. A No. 4-0 Vicryl suture is used to create a baseball stitch in a running fashion, which is then tied to compress the amnion

4.2 Patient Setup

The patient is placed supine in a standard knee arthroscopy position. The operative extremity is placed into a leg holder with a tourniquet applied to the thigh, and the nonoperative extremity is placed in a well-leg pillow.

4.3 Bone Marrow Aspiration

Before inflation of the tourniquet, a small stab incision is made just lateral to the tibial tubercle. The aspiration needle and central sharp trocar are inserted while angled proximally at 10°. A mark is made on the needle at 30 mm to avoid over-insertion. The central trocar is removed, and the first few milliliters of aspirate is discarded because of the excess amount of bone. Then, 60 mL of bone marrow is aspirated into heparinized syringes.

4.4 Mixing Bone Marrow Aspirate with Allosync Pure

After aspiration of the bone marrow, the aspirate is concentrated using the Arthrex Angel device and a total of 3 mL of the bone marrow is mixed by hand with 5 mL of the Allosync Pure. This mixture is then placed into an arthroscopic cannula delivery device. The remaining 3 mL of bone marrow concentrate is saved for later injection intra-articularly into the amnion after the graft is fixed.

4.5 ACL Technique

The tourniquet is inflated, and a standard diagnostic arthroscopy shows the ACL rupture. The allograft link sized 74 × 9.5 mm has been prepared on the back table as mentioned earlier with an adjustable button system on the tibial side and suspensory fixation BTB TightRope (Arthrex) on the femoral side. The InternalBrace (Arthrex, Naples, FL) is added to the TightRope button opposite the blue passing suture. The ACL remnants in the intercondylar notch are debrided, and a FlipCutter (Arthrex) is used to create a femoral socket through which a FiberStick (Arthrex) is placed and the suture is docked out of the lateral portal. A 12 × 4 mm PassPort cannula (Arthrex) is then placed in the medial portal. A FlipCutter is used to create the tibial socket. A TigerStick (Arthrex) and passing suture for the InternalBrace are passed through the tibia.

4.6 Suture Management and Passage

All three passing sutures are brought through the PassPort cannula medially (Fig. 3). These are docked and clamped to prevent suture bridges (Fig. 4). First, the femoral sutures are loaded into the femoral FiberStick, and the TightRope button is deployed

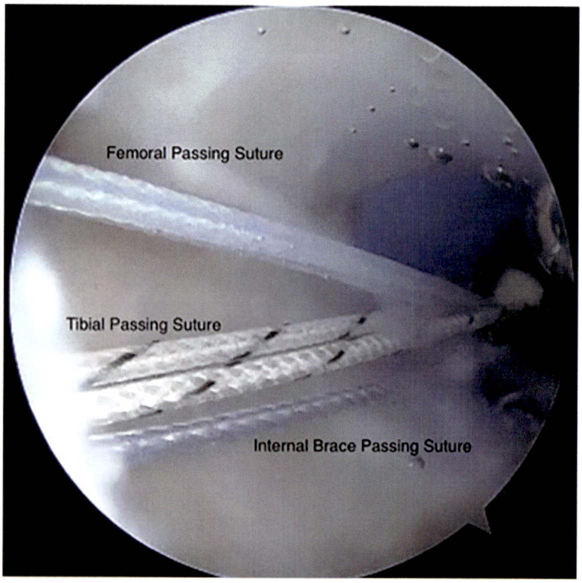

Fig. 3 Viewing from the anterolateral portal with the 30° arthroscope, the medial portal is shown with a PassPort cannula inserted and all three passing sutures retrieved

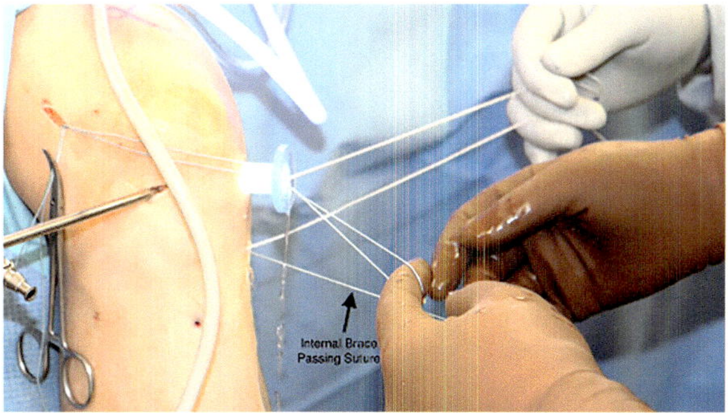

Fig. 4 Viewing outside the knee, the tibial passing sutures, InternalBrace passing sutures, and femoral passing sutures can all be seen docked

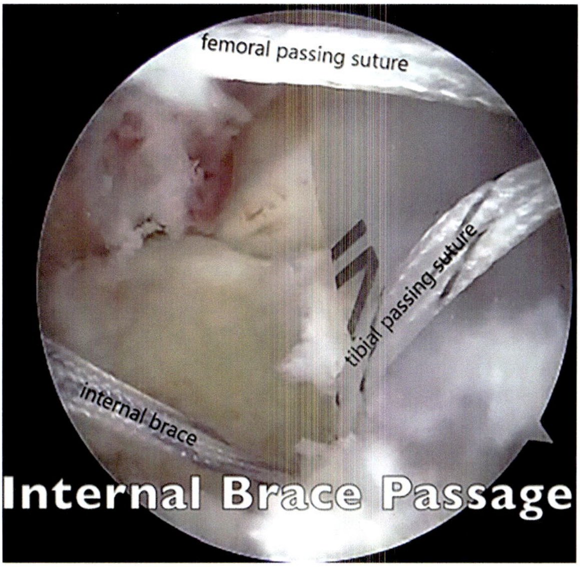

Fig. 5 Viewing from the anterolateral portal with the 30° arthroscope, the InternalBrace is being passed from the medial portal and through the tibia

on the lateral cortex of the femur. Next, the InternalBrace suture is passed through the tibia using the InternalBrace passing suture (Fig. 5).

4.7 Composite Graft Injection

By use of the arthroscopic cannula loaded with the bone marrow concentrate composite graft, we inject the graft into the femoral tunnel (Fig. 6). This is performed through the medial PassPort cannula. The delivery device is then moved to the lateral portal, and the knee is hyperflexed to inject the composite graft into the tibial tunnel (Fig. 7). The tibial graft is seen completely filling the tibial tunnel (Fig. 8).

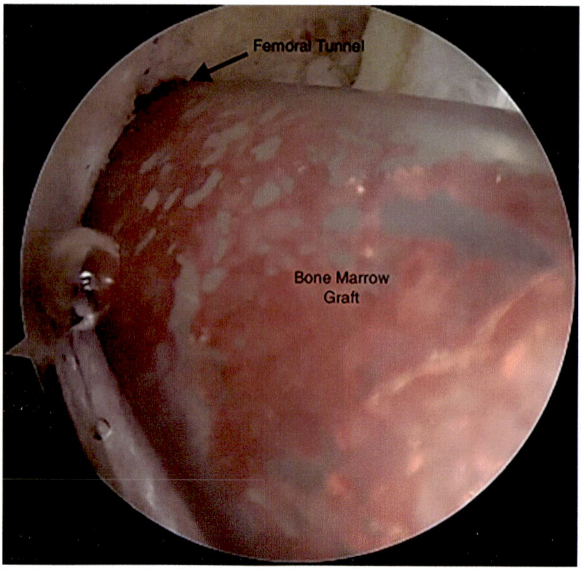

Fig. 6 Viewing from the anterolateral portal with the 30° arthroscope, the composite graft is injected into the femoral tunnel using the arthroscopic delivery cannula

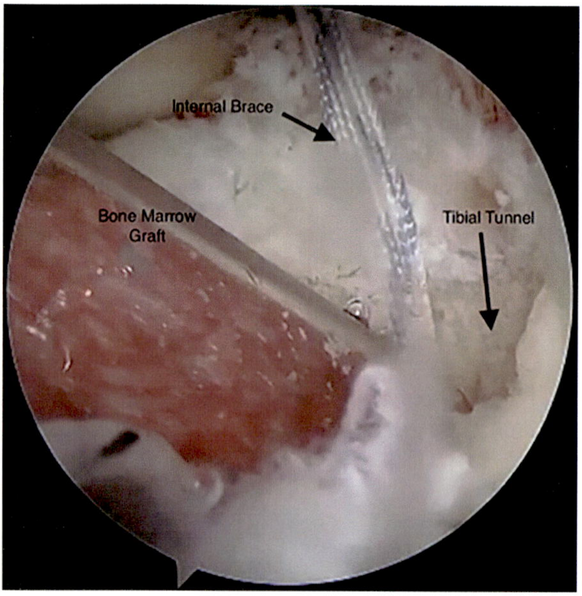

Fig. 7 Viewing from the anteromedial portal with the 30° arthroscope, the composite graft is injected into the tibial tunnel using the arthroscopic delivery cannula

4.8 ACL Graft Passage

With the white suture out of the femoral tunnel, 10 mm of femoral graft is pulled into the femur. The TigerStick sutures are then used to pass the tibia-sided sutures

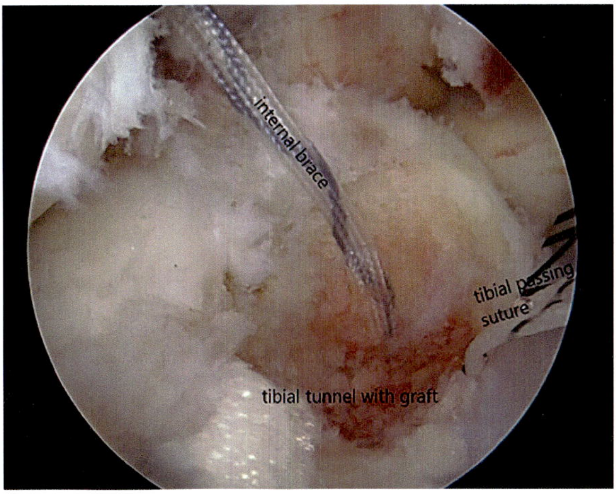

Fig. 8 Viewing from the anterolateral portal with the 30° arthroscope, the composite graft can be seen filling the tibial tunnel

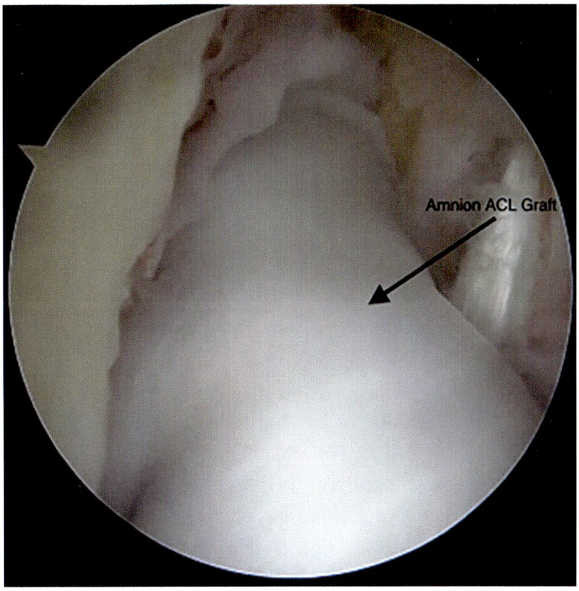

Fig. 9 Viewing from the anterolateral portal with the 30° arthroscope, the amnion anterior cruciate ligament (ACL) can be seen within the joint

through the tibia. After the tibia side of the graft is docked into the tunnel, the remaining femur-sided graft is pulled into the femur until the amnion is centered in the joint. Standard button fixation on the tibia is used at 30° of flexion of the knee (Fig. 9). The InternalBrace is then placed into a 4.75 mm SwiveLock (Arthrex) and fixed into the anterior medial tibia at full extension of the knee.

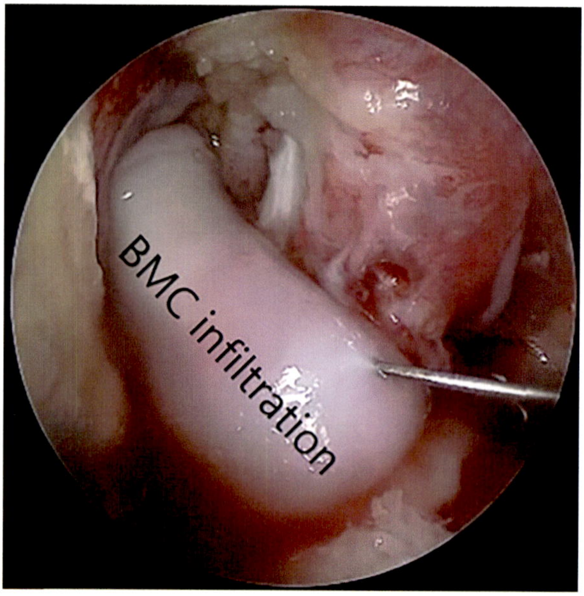

Fig. 10 Viewing from the anterolateral portal with the 30° arthroscope, the bone marrow concentrate (BMC) is seen being injected into the amnion anterior cruciate ligament

4.9 Bone Marrow Concentrate Injection

After fixation of the ACL graft, a 25-gauge needle is used to inject the remaining bone marrow concentrate into the amnion. The amnion should swell and become pink. Some small amounts of leakage from the amnion will occur (Fig. 10).

5 Rehabilitation

We use our standard ACL rehabilitation protocol. The patient is placed in a hinged knee brace locked in full extension until full quadriceps control is achieved. The patient is allowed full weight bearing in the brace immediately after surgery. In our protocol, early passive range of motion with formal physical therapy is started within the first week. The patient is then progressed through strengthening with standard ACL rehabilitation techniques.

6 Discussion

Incorporation of the graft at the tendon-to-bone interface is paramount to the success of ACL reconstructive surgery. Tunnel osteolysis has been a consistent problem regardless of graft type and remains a problem despite changing surgical techniques

[13, 14]. We recently published the Lavender technique of tunnel grafting with bone marrow concentrate and Allosync Pure [15] and the current technique combines that technique with the use of amnion. The goal of this multifactorial approach is to improve tunnel widening, overall graft incorporation, and graft vascularization which should translate to improve overall clinical outcomes.

Amniotic membrane-derived grafts have not been previously used in ACL surgery; however, the use of amnion as a biologic scaffold has been occurring for quite some time in the field of wound care and plastic surgery for complex soft-tissue regeneration [10]. The cost of the biologics may inhibit widespread use, but for patients at risk of re-rupture and for higher level athletes, this may become a great option to improve outcomes. As mentioned these biologics could be added to autograft in younger patients. There are several disadvantages and limitations to the procedure, which include extra time spent in the operating room and increased technical aspects of the procedure. The risks of this procedure include those associated with allograft use, including infection, disease transmission, and host rejection. The possibility of host rejection or reaction against the amnion is a concern, and this needs to be prospectively studied further to examine these complications. Despite those disadvantages, when combined with an allograft reconstruction and using the all-inside technique, the fertilized ACL may be the correct balance to advance rehabilitation and return to play. Together, these modalities provide an approach to improve graft incorporation in ACL reconstruction with the goal of improving clinical outcomes and decreasing graft re-rupture rates.

7 Editor's View

This technique highlights the use of amnion in ACL reconstruction [16]. One of the issues we face with ACL reconstructions is obviously the biologic environment inside the joint and amnion allows us to wrap the ACL which may lead to improved vascularization of the graft and healing of the graft at an enhanced speed. Obviously, it has its drawbacks because of the cost but with further research we may find that amnion is an important aspect of ACL reconstruction. We feel like this is the complete biologic ACL with amnion plus bone marrow concentrate in addition to grafting of the tunnels with allograft bone. This technique was developed in the middle of our evolution of biologic reconstructions which was before we started with the ability to obtain autograft bone with the graftnet. I feel this technique was an important step in our biologic ACL process and as I mentioned in the future we may see even more amnion's added to ACL grafts to improve outcomes if the studies reveal positive outcomes. Certainly if adding amnion to an allograft has the ability to improve outcomes in the allograft population that would be a dramatic development in ACL treatment.

References

1. Anderson CN, Anderson AF. Management of the anterior cruciate ligament-injured knee in the skeletally immature athlete. Clin. Sports Med. 2016;36:35–52.
2. Spindler KP, Wright RW. Clinical practice. Anterior cruciate ligament tear. N. Engl. J. Med. 2008;359:2135–42.
3. Kiapour AM, Murray MM. Basic science of anterior cruciate ligament injury and repair. Bone Joint Res. 2014;3:20–31.
4. Willadsen EM, Zahn AB, Durall CJ. What is the most effective training approach for preventing noncontact ACL injuries in high school-aged female athletes? J. Sport Rehabil. 2019;28(1):94–8.
5. Lyman S, Koulouvaris P, Sherman S, Do H, Mandl L, Marx R. Epidemiology of anterior cruciate ligament reconstruction. Trends, readmissions, and subsequent knee surgery. J. Bone Joint Surg. Am. 2009;91:2321–8.
6. Crawford SN, Waterman BR, Lubowitz JH. Long-term failure of anterior cruciate ligament reconstruction. Arthroscopy. 2013;39:1566–71.
7. Wiggins AJ, Grandhi RK, Schneider DK, Stanfield D, Webster KE, Myer GD. Risk of secondary injury in younger athletes after anterior cruciate ligament reconstruction: A systematic review and meta-analysis. Am. J. Sports Med. 2016;44:1861–76.
8. Heckmann N, Auran R, Mirzayan R. Application of amniotic tissue in orthopedic surgery. Am. J. Orthop. (Belle Mead N.J.). 2016;45:E421–5.
9. Ribon JC, Saltzman BM, Yanke AB, Cole BJ. Human amniotic membrane-derived products in sports medicine: Basic science, early results, and potential clinical applications. Am. J. Sports Med. 2016;44:2425–34.
10. Lei J, Priddy L, Lim J, Massee M, Koob T. Identification of extracellular matrix components and biological factors in micronized dehydrated human amnion/chorion membrane. Adv Wound Care (New Rochelle). 2017;6:43–53.
11. Oladeji LO, Stannard JP, Cook CR, et al. Effects of autogenous bone marrow aspirate concentrate on radiographic integration of femoral condylar osteochondral allografts. Am. J. Sports Med. 2017;45:2793–803.
12. Smith PA, Bley JA. Allograft anterior cruciate ligament reconstruction utilizing internal brace augmentation. Arthrosc. Tech. 2016;5:e1143–7.
13. Wilson TC, Kantaras A, Atay A, Johnson DL. Tunnel enlargement after anterior cruciate ligament surgery. Am. J. Sports Med. 2004;32:543–9.
14. Christensen JE, Miller MD. Knee anterior cruciate ligament injuries: Common problems and solutions. Clin. Sports Med. 2018;37:265–80.
15. Lavender C, Johnson B, Kopiec A. Augmentation of anterior cruciate ligament reconstruction with bone marrow concentrate and a suture tape. Arthrosc. Tech. 2018;7:e1289–93.
16. Lavender C, Bishop C. The fertilized anterior cruciate ligament: An all-inside anterior cruciate ligament reconstruction augmented with amnion, bone marrow concentrate, and a suture tape. Arthrosc Tech. 2019;8:e555–9.

Minimally Invasive Quad Harvest with Endoscopic Closure and Preparation with Fiber Tag Augmented Adjustable Loop Buttons

William Scott Fravel and Charles Giangarra

1 Introduction

The "all-inside" ACL reconstruction technique is a popular minimally invasive technique which has many advantages including decreased bony resection, diminished surgical trauma, decreased postoperative pain, and improved cosmesis [1]. Many variations of this technique exist, and graft options include bone-patellar tendon-bone, hamstring tendon, quadriceps tendon, and varying allograft options. The quadriceps tendon (QT) is becoming a more popular option as they can be harvested as a large diameter single bundle graft with low donor site morbidity. In addition, newer harvest instruments have made quadriceps tendon harvest far less cumbersome than previously [2]. There have been disadvantages to QT use such as quadriceps weakness and inconsistency on preparation and fixation techniques. To counteract the postoperative quadriceps weakness and donor site complications, we describe a more accurate and efficient proximal closure technique which will allow a tighter closure even through a very small incision. As we attempt to define a standardized efficient preparation technique for QT harvest, we also describe an updated technique for graft preparation which incorporates the fiber tag suture into the suspensory tightrope device and features a specialized slotted clamp.

W. S. Fravel (✉)
Department of Orthopaedic Surgery, Marshall University, Marshall University School of Medicine, Huntington, WV, USA
e-mail: Fravelw@marshall.edu

C. Giangarra
Department of Orthopaedic Surgery, VA Medical Center, Marshall University, Marshall University School of Medicine, Huntington, WV, USA
e-mail: giangarra@marshall.edu

C. Lavender (ed.), *Biologic and Nanoarthroscopic Approaches in Sports Medicine*, https://doi.org/10.1007/978-3-030-71323-2_4

2 Surgical Technique

2.1 Graft Harvest

With the patient supine and the knee flexed a small 20 mm incision is made at the distal quad from the superior border of the patella proximal. After spreading the subcutaneous tissue, the distal quad is identified. A 9 mm cutting guide is used running distal to proximal. A knife is then used to lift the distal quad off the bone and a size 0 braided suture is used to tag the quad tendon. The Graft Harvester (Arthrex Inc., Naples) is used to cut the graft proximally.

2.2 Endoscopic Closure

An arthroscope with no flow is then placed into the wound and the proximal edges of the medial and lateral quads are identified (Figs. 1, 2, and 3). A Scorpion (Arthrex Inc., Naples) device with a size 0 braided suture is used to pass a suture into the proximal medial quad. Next the inferior limb of that suture is passed through the lateral quad. This suture is then passed medial and then laterally to give a figure 8 construct. The suture is tied and cut. Distal to that a second figure of 8 construct is performed and the quad closure is tensioned and tied.

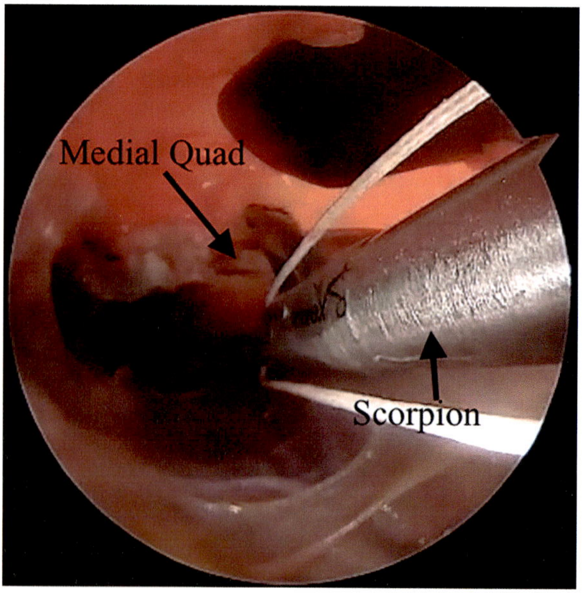

Fig. 1 The 30° arthroscope with no flow is placed into the quad incision with the right knee flexed and you can see the medial quad with the scorpion placing the first stitch

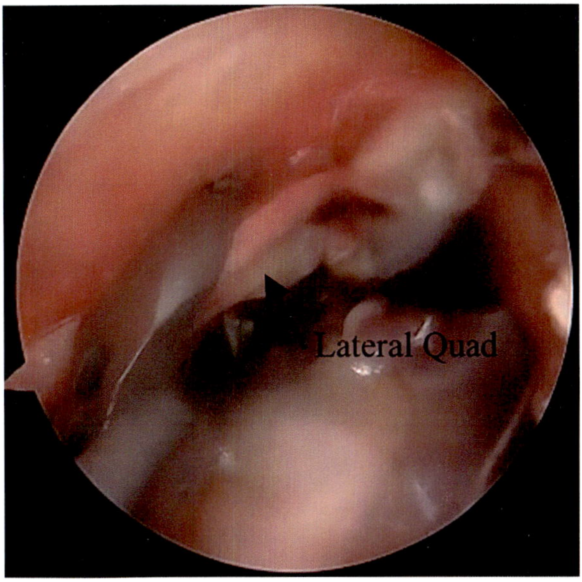

Fig. 2 The 30° arthroscope with no flow is placed into the quad incision with the right knee flexed and the lateral quad is seen with the inferior limb suture being place through the quad with the scorpion

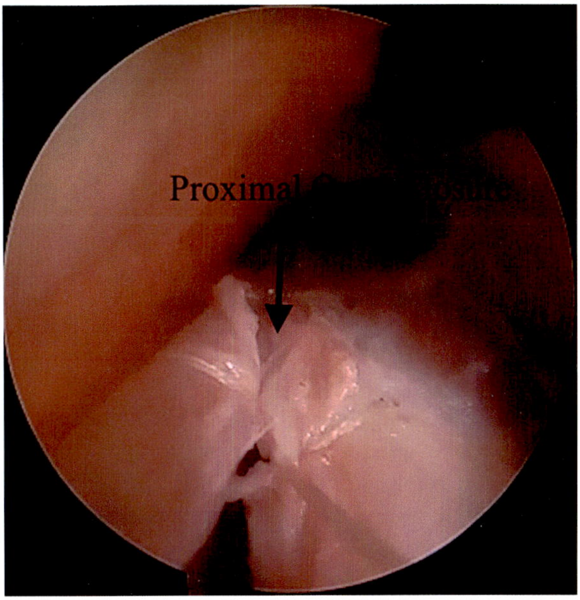

Fig. 3 The 30° arthroscope with no flow is placed into the quad incision with the right knee flexed and you can see the proximal closure of the quad is tight and approximated

2.3 Graft Preparation

The Fibertag Tightrope (Arthrex Inc., Naples) with the button superior is loaded into the inferior slot on the clamp. The inferior distal clamp is threaded through the Fibertag to secure it to the clamp with the Fibertag in the groove (Fig. 4). Care is

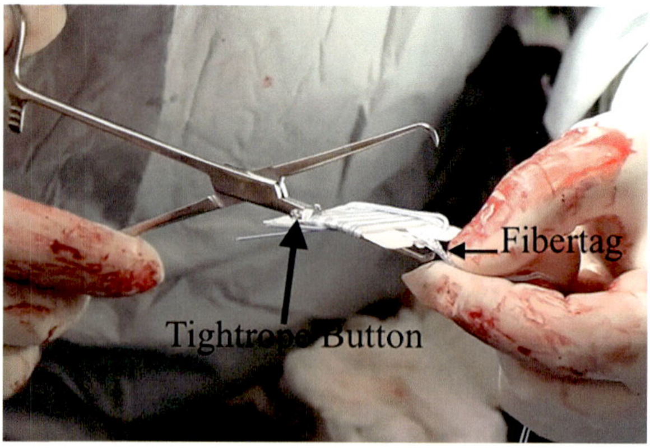

Fig. 4 The Fibertag Tightrope device is placed on the clamp with the button superior. The proximal part of the implant is placed into the inferior groove and the fibertag stitch is in the groove of the pointed clamp

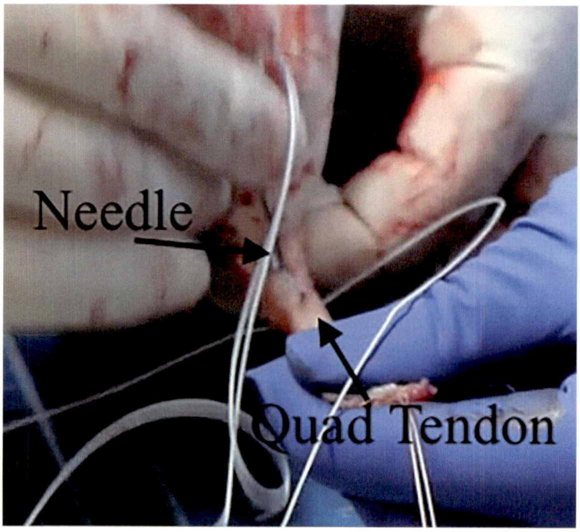

Fig. 5 The quad tendon can be seen with the needle coming through superior to inferior 25 mm from the end of the graft

taken to avoid the tightrope sutures. This construct is flipped and clamped to the last 2–3 mm of the quad. Do not place more proximal because of graft shortening. The needle is then placed superior to inferior at 25 mm into the graft (Fig. 5). Two sutures are placed superior to inferior in locking fashion with the most distal suture going through close to the clamp (Fig. 6). Next, the needle is taken up through the small opening in the construct and back down through the Firbertag (Fig. 7). Two more passes are made and the suture is cut and tied. The knot is then buried into the quad. The Fibertag ABS with the free suture superior is then placed into the clamp and tibial side of the graft is prepared in a similar fashion (Figs. 8 and 9).

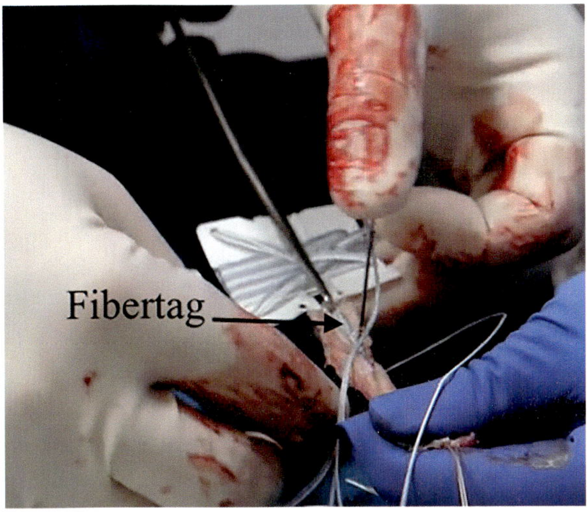

Fig. 6 The needle of the implant is seen going superior to inferior through the fibertag in the center of the graft

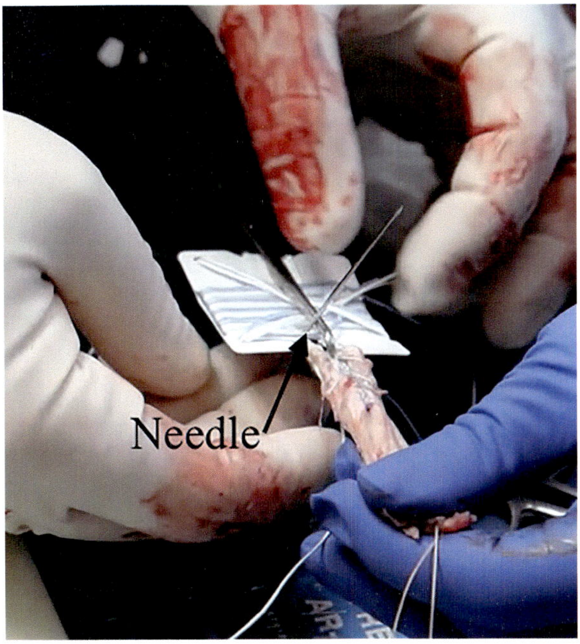

Fig. 7 The needle is seen passing through the opening in the implant card to start running distal to proximal on the graft

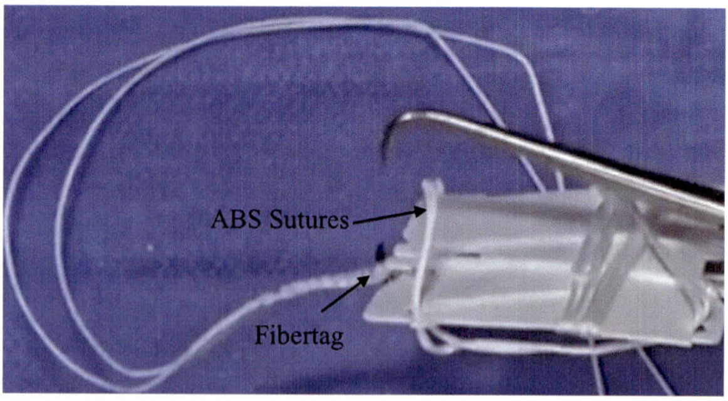

Fig. 8 The ABS Fibertag implant is placed on the clamp with the ABS sutures superior and the fiber tag through the groove on the inferior clamp

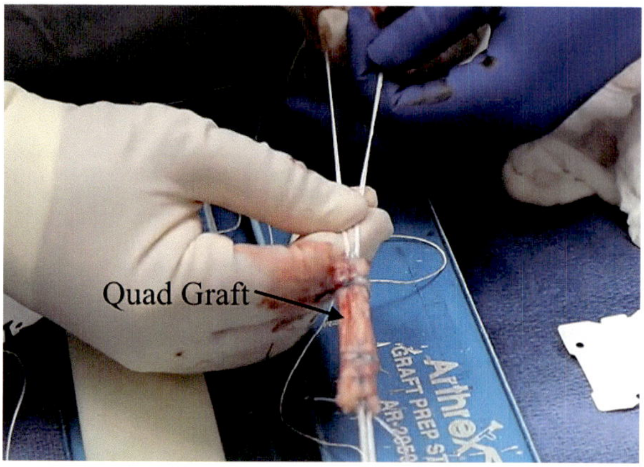

Fig. 9 The finalized Quad tendon is seen with implants on each end

3 Discussion

Current literature has continued to support the use of QT autograft and all-inside ACL reconstruction. A recent systematic review and meta-analysis demonstrated that patients with QT autograft ACL reconstruction identified similar functional outcomes and graft survival rates when compared to bone patella tendon bone (BPTB) and hamstring tendon (HT) autografts [3]. They also found significantly less harvest site pain in QT autograft patients compared to BPTB patients. When compared to ACL reconstruction with a fully drilled tibial tunnel, all-inside ACL reconstruction demonstrated no decrease in functional outcomes, and decreased postoperative pain scores in a randomized control trial [4]. Long-term follow up for QT all-inside ACL reconstruction has shown good to excellent results in both patient-reported outcome measures and functional testing [5]. The all-inside technique also has been shown to have equivalent stability testing at 2 years follow up when compared to BPTB standard reconstructions [6]. The quadriceps tendon graft has advantages including a larger cross-sectional area for a single bundle, and has been shown to have as low as a 4.2% failure rate [7].

Similar techniques have previously been described for partial thickness quadriceps tendon harvest [1, 2]. The quad tendon lends itself well for use in all-inside ACL reconstruction. Its advantages are numerous including large diameter and consistency of the graft. Performing the harvest from a minimally invasive incision is possible; however, closure 7 cm proximal for optimal graft length can be difficult through the smaller incisions. The closure technique we describe here has the cosmetic advantage of using a small incision and still ensuring a tight proximal closure which may prevent quadriceps weakness postoperatively. Although the endoscopic closure allows a better closure through a small incision, it does add cost to the case (Table 1). The updated Fiber Tag Tightrope and ABS devices used for graft preparation when added to the new slotted clamp improve the efficiency and security of the graft preparation when compared to previous methods. In the technique described here we believe the strength, security, and reproducibility of the preparation will improve. Pearls of the technique are that the button and free sutures should face superiorly when the implant is added into the slotted clamp. When coming inferior to superior through the card you need to pass through the opening in the card. Care should be taken not to clamp the QT graft too far distally which can lead to shortening of the graft (Table 2). Overall both techniques described here are easily reproducible and with careful attention should lead to improved all-inside ACL reconstruction outcomes.

Table 1 Advantages and disadvantages of proximal endoscopic closure

Advantages
Ability to visualize your proximal closure even through a smaller incision
Faster closure with the Scorpion (Arthrex Inc, Naples)
Disadvantages
Cost of the Scorpion and needle
Additional time to load the Scorpion
Learning curve for surgeons not familiar with the Scorpion

Table 2 Pearls and pitfalls of graft preparation

Pearls
Tightrope button and free ABS stitches should be superior when implant placed into the clamp
Clamp is turned upside down before placing onto the quad
First stitch should be 25 CM from the end of the graft
Tension each stitch independently
Pitfalls
Care should be taken not to clamp the quad to far proximal which would shorten the graft
When coming inferior to superior at end of the graft the suture must go through space in card

4 Editor's View

This technique improves the harvest and preparation of the quad tendon graft for ACL reconstruction. We have started using the QT as our primary ACL graft and the combination of this harvest and preparation has helped our efficiency and outcomes. The closure has allowed our incisions to become smaller and the overall harvest to become more minimally invasive. This has been very noticeable in patients postoperative recovery and we have seen a noticeable improvement in their quadriceps strength postoperatively. Obviously being able to harvest the graft through a smaller incision improves cosmetic results. The development of the clamp and fiber tag loaded implants has had an improvement on the speed of our ability to prepare the graft and in my opinion improves the consistency of the graph and stability of the graft. This cut our preparation time down in half. I fully believe that it is worth opening the scorpion device to provide the closure proximally and also utilize the fiber attack-loaded implants when doing quadriceps tendon preparation.

References

1. Slone HS, Ashford WB, Xerogeanes JW. Minimally invasive quadriceps tendon harvest and graft preparation for all-inside anterior cruciate ligament reconstruction. Arthrosc. Tech. 2016;5(5):e1049–56. Published 2016 Sep 19. https://doi.org/10.1016/j.eats.2016.05.012.
2. Sprowls G, Robin B. The quad link technique for an all-soft-tissue quadriceps graft in minimally invasive, all-inside anterior cruciate ligament reconstruction. Arthrosc. Tech. 2018;7(8):e845–52.
3. Mouarbes D, Menetrey J, Marot V, Courtot L, Berard E, Cavaignac E. Anterior cruciate ligament reconstruction: A systematic review and meta-analysis of outcomes for quadriceps tendon autograft versus bone-patellar tendon-bone and hamstring-tendon autografts. Am. J. Sports Med. 2019;47(14):3531–40. https://doi.org/10.1177/0363546518825340.
4. Lubowitz JH, Schwartzberg R, Smith P. Randomized controlled trial comparing all-inside anterior cruciate ligament reconstruction technique with anterior cruciate ligament reconstruction with a full tibial tunnel. Arthroscopy. 2013;29(7):1195–200. https://doi.org/10.1016/j.arthro.2013.04.009.
5. Galan H, Escalante M, Vedova F, Slullitel D. All inside full thickness quadriceps tendon ACL reconstruction: Long term follow up results. J Exp Orthop. 2020 December;7:13.
6. Smith P, Cook C, Bley J. All-inside quadrupled semitendinosus autograft shows stability equivalent to patellar tendon autograft anterior cruciate ligament reconstruction: Randomized controlled trial in athletes 24 years or younger. Arthroscopy. 2020;36(6):P1629–46.
7. Xerogeanes J. Quadriceps tendon graft for anterior cruciate ligament reconstruction: The graft of the future. Arthroscopy. 2019;35(3):696–7.

The Lavender Fertilized Anterior Cruciate Ligament Reconstruction: A Quadriceps Tendon All-Inside Reconstruction Fertilized with Bone Marrow Concentrate, Demineralized Bone Matrix, and Autograft Bone

Baylor Blickenstaff and Chad Lavender

1 Introduction

This chapter focuses on showing how our unique biologic composite is obtained and then added back into the tunnels on both the femoral and tibial sides during a quadriceps tendon, all-inside anterior cruciate ligament reconstruction [1]. In previous chapters, we have revealed our biologic composite, but in this chapter, we add autograft bone and perform a quad tendon all-inside ACL reconstruction. The all-inside ACL reconstruction was first described by Lubowitz in 2006, first as a trans-tibial drilling of both tunnels, and has since evolved to outside-in drilling of both femoral and tibial tunnels. Graft re-rupture rates of ACL reconstruction with all techniques have been reported as high as 11% [2], and secondary ACL injury rates to either the operative or contralateral side have been reported as 23% in athletes under the age of 25 [3]. These numbers are concerning and despite bone-patellar tendon-bone reconstruction being the current gold standard, our field is constantly investigating new methods to attempt to decrease these devastating complications. Bone marrow concentrate has been used in orthopedics to aid in the healing of

With permission from Arthroscopy Techniques Lavender C, Bishop C. The Fertilized Anterior Cruciate Ligament: An All-Inside Anterior Cruciate Ligament Reconstruction Augmented with Amnion, Bone Marrow Concentrate, and a Suture Tape. *Arthroscopic Techniques* 2019; 8: e555–e559.

B. Blickenstaff
Department of Orthopaedic Surgery, Marshall University, Scott Depot, WV, USA
e-mail: Blickenstafb@marshall.edu

C. Lavender (✉)
Orthopaedic Surgery Sports Medicine, Marshall University, Scott Depot, WV, USA

C. Lavender (ed.), *Biologic and Nanoarthroscopic Approaches in Sports Medicine*, https://doi.org/10.1007/978-3-030-71323-2_5

injuries such as avascular necrosis and osteochondral lesions [4]. Recently, a technique was developed using bone marrow concentrate and suture tape augmentation for bone-patella tendon-bone grafts [5]. We have begun to use predominantly quadriceps autografts for our reconstructions. So it was necessary to create this technique to incorporate biologics and the internal brace into the reconstruction.

This technique is the first described which augments an ACL reconstructions with bone marrow concentrate and autograft bone collected from the femoral and tibial tunnel reamings via GraftNet Autologous Tissue Collector (Arthrex). Bone marrow concentrate has been used in many other orthopedic conditions with good results. Autograft bone combined with Allosync (Arthrex) demineralized bone matrix is used to aid in graft incorporation and aims to prevent graft re-rupture due to the osteogenic, osteoinductive, and osteoconductive nature of autograft. Collecting autograft reamings from the tunnels also decreases the amount of allograft needed for the composite graft, decreasing overall cost as well as providing a more native biochemical graft. We augment our reconstruction with suture tape, which has been shown to reduce the elongation of the graft and increase ultimate load-to-failure [6]. Furthermore, the suture tape does not stress-shield the graft which allows the graft to support the knee without weakening in the long run.

By utilizing this all-inside technique, we are able to perform anatomic reconstruction of the ACL with augmented fixation of the graft with suture tape, and we hypothesize that by adding BMC with allograft demineralized bone matrix and autograft bone the tunnels will fill in quicker allowing a stronger construct that can decrease re-rupture rates.

2 Indications

Patients with an ACL tear which are active, young, and have an interest to return to the highest level of competition.

3 Contraindications

Previous quadricep harvest: In patients with previous quadriceps harvest using a contralateral quadriceps graft is a great option.

4 Surgical Technique

4.1 Patient Setup

The patient is placed supine in a standard knee arthroscopy position. The operative extremity is placed into a leg holder with a tourniquet applied to the thigh, and the contralateral extremity is placed into a well-padded leg pillow. The operative extremity is prepped and draped in the usual fashion.

4.2 Bone Marrow Aspiration

Before inflating the tourniquet, a small stab incision is made just lateral to the tibial tubercle. A Jamshidi needle (Arthrex) and central sharp trocar are inserted at a 10° angle proximally. We make a mark on the needle at 30 mm to avoid over insertion. Then, 60 cc of bone marrow is aspirated into heparinized syringes. This aspiration is then concentrated using the Arthrex Angel System into 5 cc of bone marrow concentrate.

4.3 ACL Technique

The tourniquet is inflated, and a standard diagnostic arthroscopy confirms the ACL rupture. A standard quadriceps tendon graft harvest is performed to achieve a graft length of 66 mm of all soft tissue. FiberTag (Arthrex) is then used to prepare the quadriceps into an all-inside construct. The femoral side has a TightRope RT (Arthrex), while the tibial side has an attachable button system (Arthrex) added. The TightRope system should be loosened to add more length so that the button on the femur can later be flipped and still leave space to inject the bone marrow graft into the femur before bringing the graft into the joint. At this point, after loosening the system, the suture tape (InternalBrace, Arthrex) is placed through the button in a reinforcement fashion. The remnants of the ACL are debrided, and the FlipCutter (Arthrex) is used to make a 30 mm femoral socket in the standard location.

4.4 Femoral Socket Preparation and Autograft Collection

An aggressive shaver with the GraftNet applied is placed through the lateral portal just under the FlipCutter (Fig. 1). The shaver is turned on, and the FlipCutter drills the socket in a retrograde fashion (Fig. 2). After the socket is created, the water is turned off and the GraftNet is inserted into a Frazier-tip suction (Conmed, Utica,

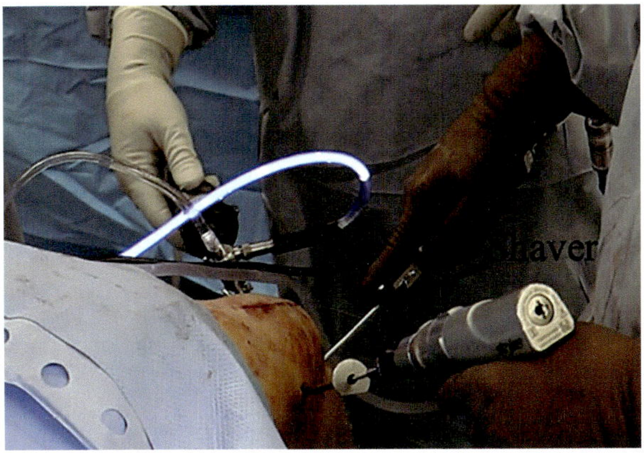

Fig. 1 The right knee is flexed and the patient is supine. The shaver with the GraftNet (Arthrex) applied to the suction has been placed into the lateral portal, while the FlipCutter (Arthrex) can be seen creating the femoral tunnel. The 30° arthroscope has been placed into the medial portal

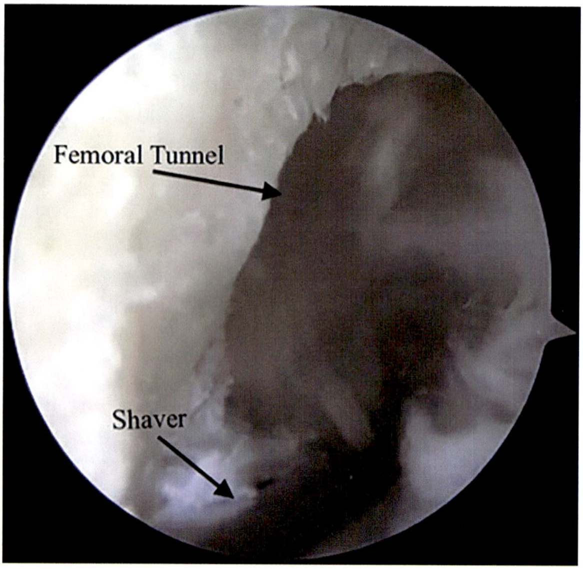

Fig. 2 A view from the 30° arthroscope placed in the medial portal shows the femoral tunnel being reamed. The shaver with the GraftNet(Arthrex) applied has been placed inferior to the femoral tunnel and obtains autograft bone

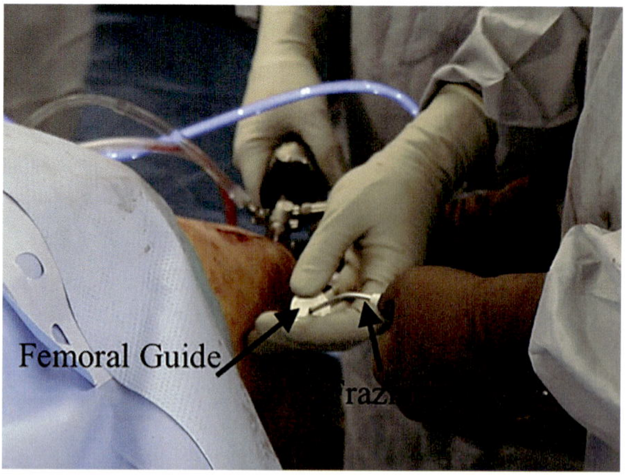

Fig. 3 The right knee is flexed and the patient is supine. A view from outside the joint shows a Frazier suction tip placed through the femoral guide; the arthroscope is placed in the medial portal

NY) and replaces the FlipCutter in the guide (Figs. 3 and 4). Flow is then turned back on. After making the femoral socket, a no.2 FiberStick (Arthrex) is introduced into the joint and docked outside the lateral portal until the tibial tunnel is completed.

4.5 Tibial Tunnel Socket Preparation and Autograft Bone Collection

The tibial tunnel is also created with the FlipCutter, and the shaver with GraftNet applied is placed through the medial portal while drilling (Fig. 5). Again, the

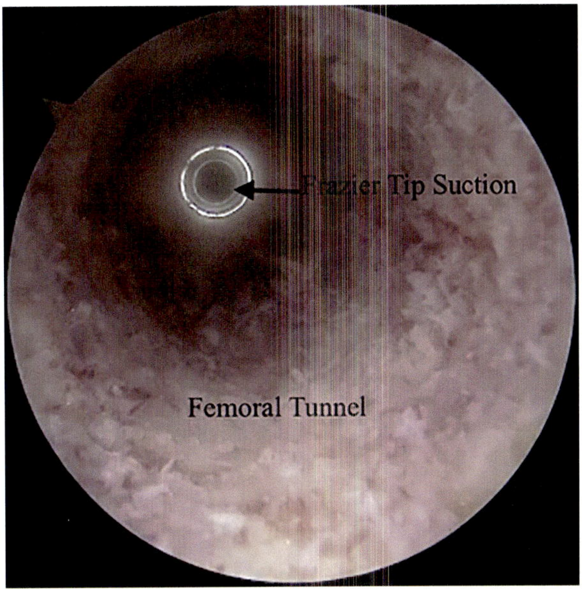

Fig. 4 A view from the medial portal with the 30° arthroscope into the femoral tunnel shows the Frazier suction tip within the guide; all reamed bone has been removed from the tunnel

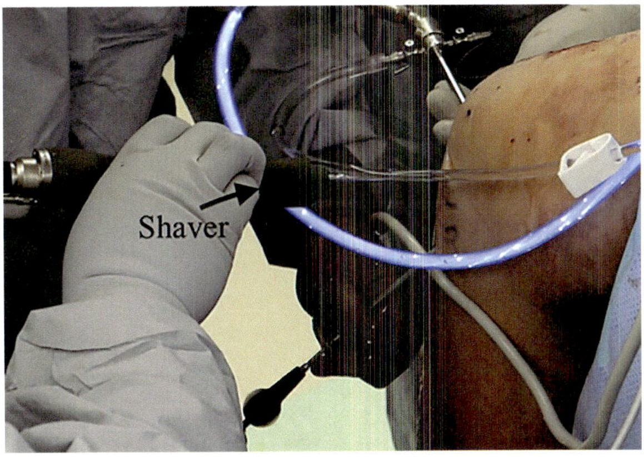

Fig. 5 The right knee is flexed and the patient is supine. A view from outside of the joint shows the tibia reamed with the FlipCutter; the shaver with GraftNet (Arthrex) has been placed through the medial portal while viewing from the lateral portal with the 30° arthroscope

Frazier-tip suction can be used with the GraftNet up through the guide. A second passing FiberStick is passed through the tibia, and both sutures are brought out medially. The TightRope is then passed into the joint in the standard fashion and brought out of the femur and flipped on the lateral cortex.

4.6 Mixing Bone Marrow Aspiration with AlloSync Pure

The aspirated bone marrow is concentrated using the Arthrex Angel device. We collected 4 cc of autograft bone, which is mixed with 5 cc of AlloSync Pure (Arthrex)

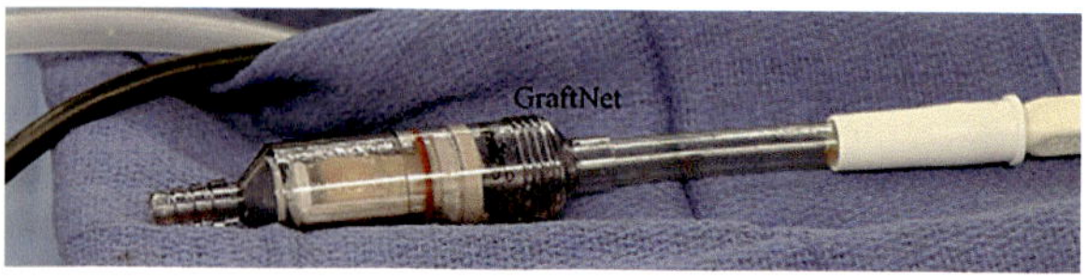

Fig. 6 The GraftNet (Arthrex) can be seen with bone graft within the cartridge

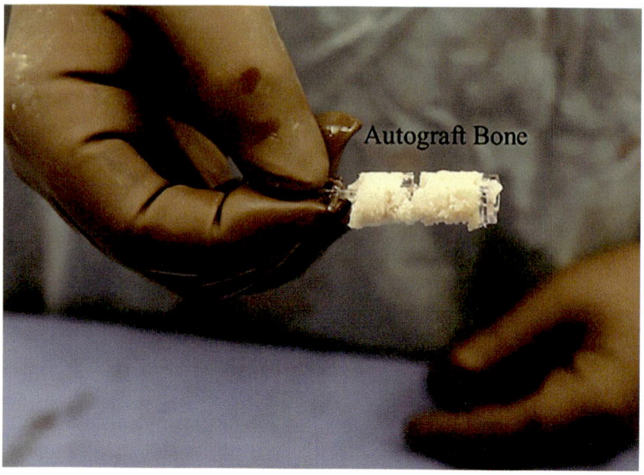

Fig. 7 The inner sleeve can be seen after being removed from the GraftNet (Arthrex); it contains the collected autograft bone

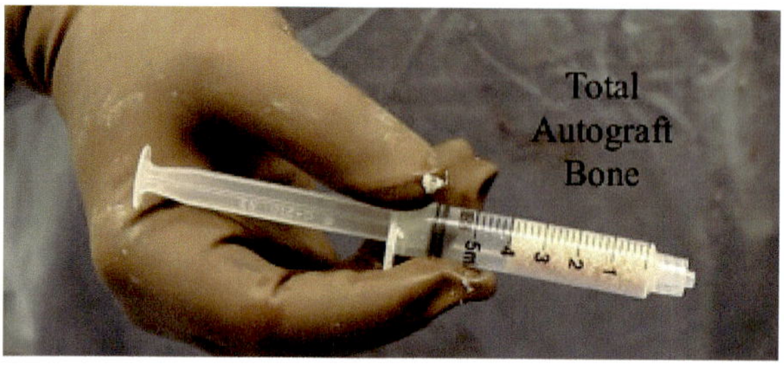

Fig. 8 Autograft bone is transferred to a small syringe to give an accurate calculation of the amount, which in this case was 4 cc

(Figs. 6, 7, and 8). This mixture is added to 5 cc of bone marrow concentrate (Fig. 9), and the resulting mixture is then placed into an arthroscopic cannula device.

4.7 Bone Marrow Graft Passage

The arthroscopic cannula is placed through the medial portal, and the knee is hyper-flexed. The graft is injected into the femoral tunnel to fill the entire tunnel (Figs. 10 and 11). The delivery cannula is then placed from the lateral portal and down into the tibia, and the tibial tunnel is completely filled with the composite graft (Figs. 12 and 13).

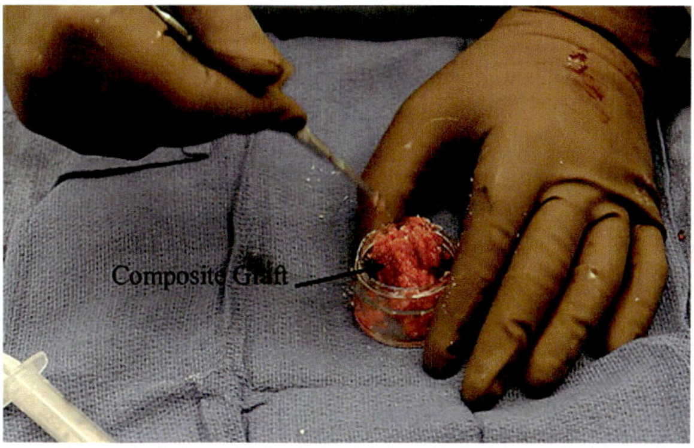

Fig. 9 The mixture of bone marrow concentrate and AlloSync Pure (Arthrex) with autograft bone being mixed by hand

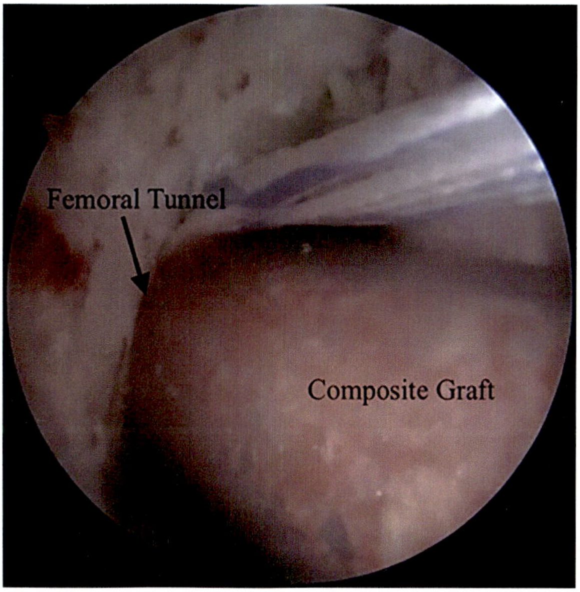

Fig. 10 Viewing from the lateral portal with a 30° arthroscope, the delivery cannula is placed through the medial portal and can be seen while the composite graft is injected into the femoral tunnel

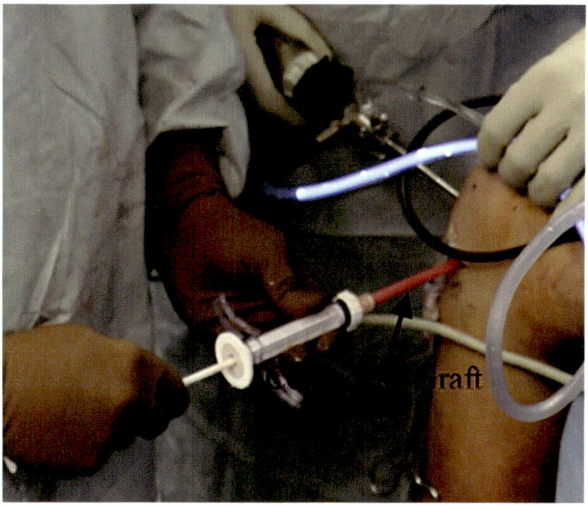

Fig. 11 The right knee is flexed and the patient is supine. A view from outside the joint shows the composite graft being injected into the femoral tunnel from the medial portal

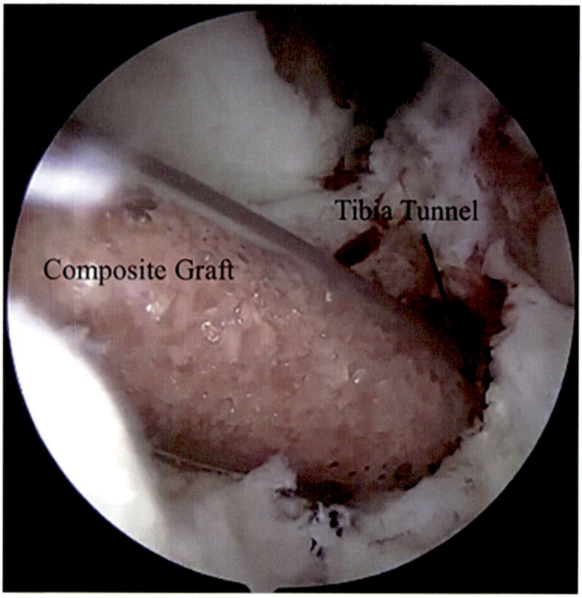

Fig. 12 A view from the medial portal with a 30° arthroscope shows the delivery device placed through the lateral portal and the composite graft being injected into the tibial tunnel

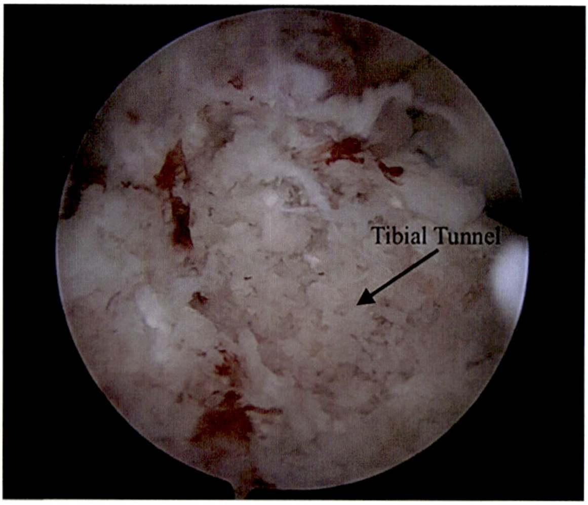

Fig. 13 A view from the lateral portal with a 30° arthroscope shows the tibial tunnel completely filled with the composite graft mixture

4.8 Graft Passage

Ten millimeters of the femoral side of the graft is then delivered into the femur, and the tibial tails are then "dunked" along with the internal brace sutures. The graft is tensioned on each side. The attachable button system is then secured on the tibia with a 12 mm button. Once the graft is fixed, the internal brace is placed into a

4.75 mm SwivelLock (Arthrex) anchor, which is placed in standard fashion on the anteromedial tibia with the leg in full extension.

5 Rehabilitation

We use our standard ACL rehabilitation protocol. The patient is placed in a hinged knee brace locked in the full extension until full quadriceps control is achieved. The patient is allowed full weight bearing in the brace immediately after surgery. In our protocol, early passive range of motion with formal physical therapy is started within the first week. The patient is then progressed through strengthening with standard ACL rehabilitation techniques.

6 Discussion

The all-inside ACL reconstruction technique has shown equivalent functional outcomes and decreased visual analog pain scores compared to reconstruction using a full tibial tunnel [7]. We have augmented our all-inside technique with the harvesting of autologous graft from tunnel reamings and creation of a composite graft using bone marrow concentrate and AlloSync Pure. We hypothesize that this composite graft, when injected into the femoral and tibial tunnels after graft insertion, could accelerate graft incorporation, decrease tunnel widening, and hopefully decrease early re-rupture rates. Early imaging shown in Figs. 14 and 15 leads to the excitement our hypothesis is correct (Fig. 14). Harvesting of the bone marrow concentrate and autologous bone graft is simple and does not add a significant amount of length to the overall operative time, as the bone marrow concentrate harvest at the proximal tibia is close to the operative site and is already prepped out. The GraftNet attaches to the standard Arthrex shaver and collects the reamings as the tunnels are drilled. The local autograft that we recover allows us to use a smaller volume of demineralized bone matrix, helping to decrease costs while theoretically improving the biologic properties of the graft mixture. Also, the use of autograft eliminates the risk of disease or tissue reaction associated with allograft.

There are a few important technical pearls of this technique that are worth discussing. First, it is imperative to use a Frazier suction tip to maximize the volume of autologous bone graft collected from tunnel reamings. After collecting the reamings via the GraftNet on the femoral side, we like to detach the GraftNet, empty the autograft into a container on the back table, and reattach the GraftNet for tibial reamings collection. This prevents the device from clogging due to too high a volume of graft in the collector.

Limitations of this technique include a theoretical risk of donor-site morbidity at the bone marrow harvesting site. However, the site of aspiration is in the sterile field, the needle used to aspirate is small, and we mark 30 mm on the needle as to not insert too deeply. We have performed 100 aspirations in this manner with no

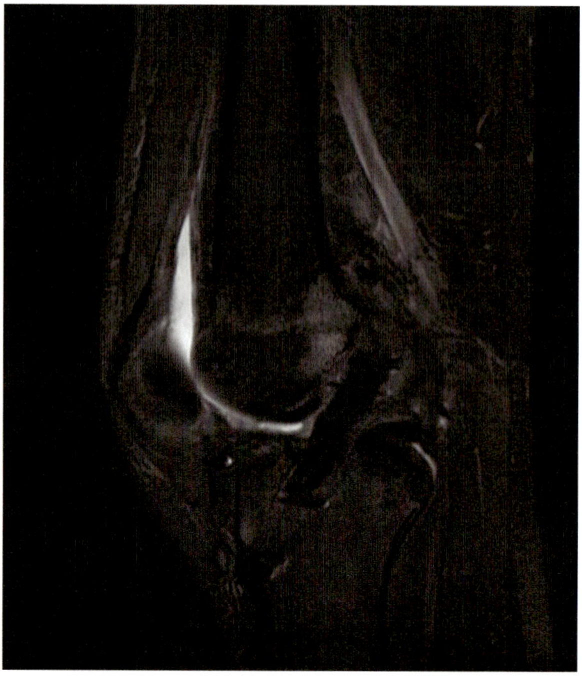

Fig. 14 A sagittal MRI status post surgery at 9 weeks showing excellent graft consistency and incorporation of the tibial socket at the base of the tunnel

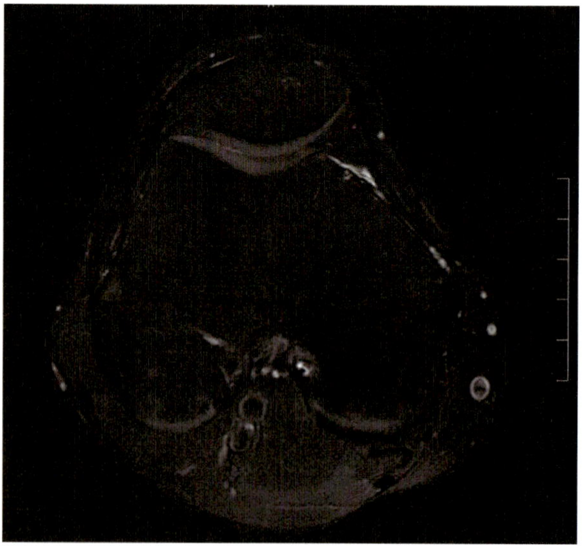

Fig. 15 An axial MRI image status post surgery at 2 years with complete consolidation of the femoral tunnel

tibial donor site morbidity. Another limitation could be the inherent difficulty of the all-inside reconstruction technique compared to standard ACL reconstruction; however, with equivalent functional outcomes and decreased VAS scores, we prefer the all-inside technique. There is a cost associated with using the GraftNet; however, this cost may be offset by the reduced usage of demineralized bone matrix due to a larger collection of autograft bone. Bone-patellar tendon-bone ACL reconstruction is still the gold standard; however, we are optimistic especially with the above imaging that the all-inside technique augmented with our composite graft of bone marrow concentrate, autologous bone graft, and AlloSync Pure can lead to fewer early graft re-ruptures which are devastating to athletes.

7 Editor's View

In regards to ACL reconstruction, I feel this technique allows us to use the most up to date enhanced biologic tools such as the GraftNet in addition to Allosync Pure and BMC. Add in the internal brace and I feel that this is the most up-to-date innovative technique for ACL reconstructions we have had in a long time. The fact that we are able to take autograft bone and utilize that in our fertilization process has really improved our technique from a cellular standpoint. With the increased attention toward quad tendon autografts, this technique is a great way to use that graft and also next-generation biologics. The quad tendon being a soft tissue graft makes it easy to fertilize both tunnels and also add our internal brace all of this being performed in an all inside fashion. Our retrospective review of the first 16 patients with The Fertilized ACL showed at 2 years an IKDC score of 81/87, no re-ruptures, no infections, and a very high return to pre-operative activity. We are closely monitoring our results in our prospective clinical trial and look forward to comparing this against a gold standard BTB autograft in the future. I personally feel this is a graft and technique that can be used for any athlete of any caliber and had been very pleased with the results and their return to activity status. We use it in 100% of our young and active patients.

References

1. Lavender C, Johnson B, Singh V, Dennis E, Torres L. The Lavender fertilized anterior cruciate ligament reconstruction: a quadriceps tendon all-inside reconstruction fertilized with bone marrow concentrate, demineralized bone matrix, and autograft bone. Arthrosc Tech. 2019;8:e1019–23.
2. Crawford SN, Waterman BR, Lubowitz JH. Long-term failure of anterior cruciate ligament reconstruction. Arthroscopy. 2013;39:1566–71.
3. Wiggins AJ, Grandhi RK, Schneider DK, Stanfield D, Webster KE, Myer GD. Risk of secondary injury in younger athletes after anterior cruciate ligament reconstruction: a systematic review and meta-analysis. Am. J. Sports Med. 2016;44:1861–76.
4. Imam MA, Mahmoud SSS, Holton J, Abouelmaati D, Elsherbini Y, Snow M. A systematic review of the concept and clinical applications of bone marrow aspirate concentrate in orthopaedics. SICOT J. 2017;3:17.
5. Lavender C, Johnson B, Kopiec A. Augmentation of anterior cruciate ligament reconstruction with bone marrow concentrate and a suture tape. Arthrosc Tech. 2018;7:e1289–93.
6. Bachmaier S, Smith PA, Bley J, Wijdicks CA. Independent suture tape reinforcement of small and standard diameter grafts for anterior cruciate ligament reconstruction: a biomechanical full construct model. Arthroscopy. 2018;34(2):490–9.
7. Lubowitz JH, Schwartzberg R, Smith P. Randomized controlled trial comparing all-inside anterior cruciate ligament reconstruction technique with anterior cruciate ligament reconstruction with a full tibial tunnel. Arthroscopy. 2013;29:1195–200.

The ACT Procedure: Autograft Cartilage Transfer Using an Autologous Tissue Collector

Syed Ali Sina Adil and Chad Lavender

1 Introduction

Articular cartilage defects of the knee are a common cause of knee pain and dysfunction. Although the exact etiology is unknown, a number of causes have been proposed, including trauma, vascular insults, genetics, and endocrinopathies [1]. Of these mechanisms, repetitive trauma has been thought to be the primary cause due to its primary location on the lateral aspect of the medial femoral condyle, which may encounter a hypertrophic tibial spine [2]. In the past few decades, advances in arthroscopy and magnetic resonance imaging (MRI) have led to an increased rate of detection of articular defects of the knee [3]. The exact prevalence of osteochondral lesions is unknown; studies have reported rates of 15–29 cases per 100,000 persons [4]. Because of the poor healing potential of hyaline cartilage, articular defects may lead to premature osteoarthritis with significant impairment in function and quality of life. Initial imaging consists of plain radiographs including anteroposterior, tunnel, lateral, and merchant views. Plain radiographs help to localize lesions, determine the size, and evaluate the status of the distal femoral physis in adolescents. MRI is often the imaging modality of choice because of its ability to show lesions that are not evident on plain radiographs [1]. Initial treatment options include nonoperative management with activity modification, nonsteroidal anti-inflammatory drugs, and intra-articular corticosteroids. However, osteochondral lesions in adults typically have an unremitting course with progressive dysfunction and impairment. Surgical options for unstable lesions and those in which conservative measures fail include arthroscopic drilling, debridement and bone grafting, internal fixation, microfracture, autologous

S. A. S. Adil
PGY3 Marshall University, Scott Depot, WV, USA
e-mail: adil@marshall.edu

C. Lavender (✉)
Orthopaedic Surgery Sports Medicine, Marshall University, Scott Depot, WV, USA

C. Lavender (ed.), *Biologic and Nanoarthroscopic Approaches in Sports Medicine*, https://doi.org/10.1007/978-3-030-71323-2_6

chondrocyte implantation (ACI), and osteochondral autograft and allograft. Of these techniques, ACI which involves the regeneration of hyaline cartilage through a 2-stage procedure has been used to treat large articular defects with minimal donor-site morbidity. To circumvent the 2-stage ACI, newer techniques aim to achieve the clinical results of ACI with a 1-step process. We present a technique for a single-stage autologous chondrocyte transplantation procedure using the GraftNet tissue collector (Arthrex, Naples, FL). This is a 1-step surgical approach that combines bone marrow concentrate, healthy autologous hyaline tissue, and allograft BioCartilage (Arthrex) as a scaffold to treat particular defects of the knee. With permission Lavender et al. Autograft Cartilage Transfer Augmented with bone marrow concentrate and allograft extracellular matrix. Arthroscopic Techniques 2020;9:e199-e203.

2 Indications

Indications for this procedure include small contained lesions which are amenable to cartilage transfer techniques. This would include those lesions less than 4 cm^2. This is also indicated in patients who have failed standard microfracture techniques.

3 Contraindications

Contradindication for this technique include large lesions typically treated with osteochondral allografts or large structural autograft transfers. Lesions with bone loss and lesions in older patients more amenable to reconstruction techniques would also be contradindications.

4 Surgical Technique

4.1 Patient Setup

The patient is placed supine in a standard knee arthroscopy position. The operative extremity is placed into a leg holder with a tourniquet applied to the thigh, and the nonoperative extremity is placed in a well-padded leg pillow. Skin is prepped in the usual sterile technique.

4.2 Bone Marrow Aspiration

Before the tourniquet is inflated, a small stab incision is made just lateral to the tibial tubercle. An aspiration needle and central sharp trocar are inserted proximally at approximately a 10-degree angle. A mark is made on the needle at 30 mm to avoid over-insertion. Then, 60 mL of bone marrow is aspirated into heparinized syringes. This aspirated material is concentrated using the Arthrex Angel System to 5 mL of bone marrow concentrate.

4.3 Autograft Cartilage Transfer Technique

The tourniquet is inflated, and a standard diagnostic arthroscopy reveals the large osteochondral defect in the lateral femoral condyle (Figs. 1 and 2). The lesion is

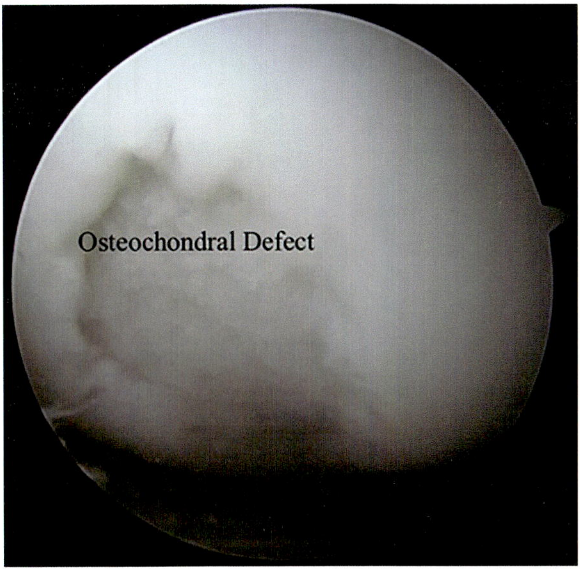

Fig. 1 With the patient supine, the right knee in 90 of flexion, and the arthroscope placed through the medial portal, the large osteochondral lesion on the lateral femoral condyle can be seen

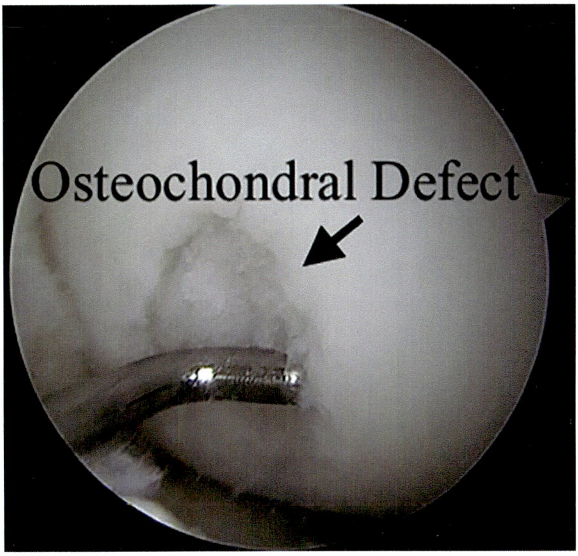

Fig. 2 With the patient supine, the right knee in 90 of flexion, and the arthroscope placed through the medial portal, a standard probe is applied to the large osteochondral lesion on the lateral femoral condyle

prepared and debrided using a shaver and then a small curette. After the lesion has been prepared, a standard microfracture technique is performed with a small drilling device (PowerPick; Arthrex). Circumferential perforations are created first, followed by central perforations to a bleeding base (Figs. 3 and 4).

Next, the harvesting process is begun. With the knee in full extension, the arthroscope is inserted into the lateral portal and a shaver with the GraftNet device applied

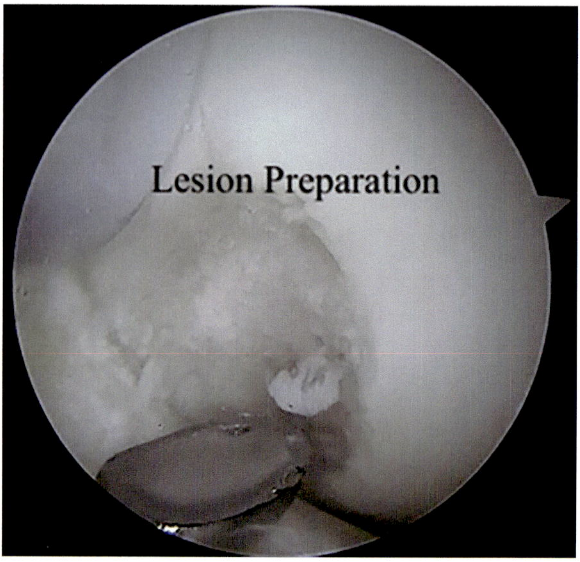

Fig. 3 With the patient supine, the right knee in 90 of flexion, and the arthroscope placed through the medial portal, a curette is used to prepare the large osteochondral lesion on the lateral femoral condyle

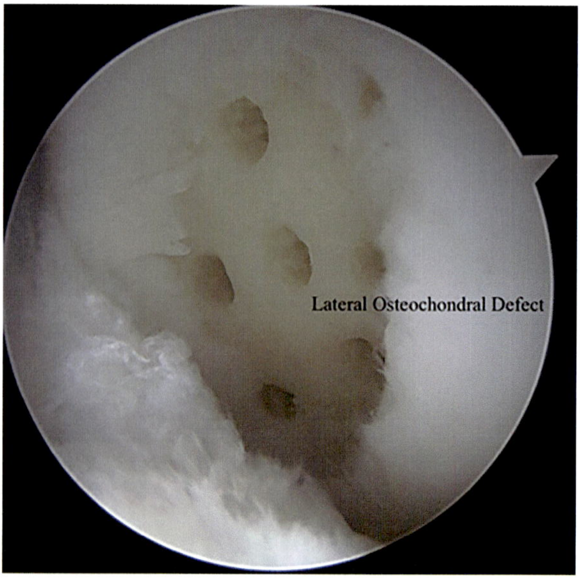

Fig. 4 With the patient supine, the right knee in 90 of flexion, and the arthroscope placed through the medial portal, the large osteochondral lesion on the lateral femoral condyle has been prepared; a microfracture is seen on the lesion surface

is placed through the medial portal. Prior to harvesting, it is important to debride as much synovium as possible from the areas of harvesting to increase the amount of pure cartilage harvested. The shaver is then used to harvest the non-articulating portion of cartilage from the medial femur (Figs. 5 and 6). The shaver and arthroscope are switched, and in similar fashion, autograft cartilage is harvested from the lateral

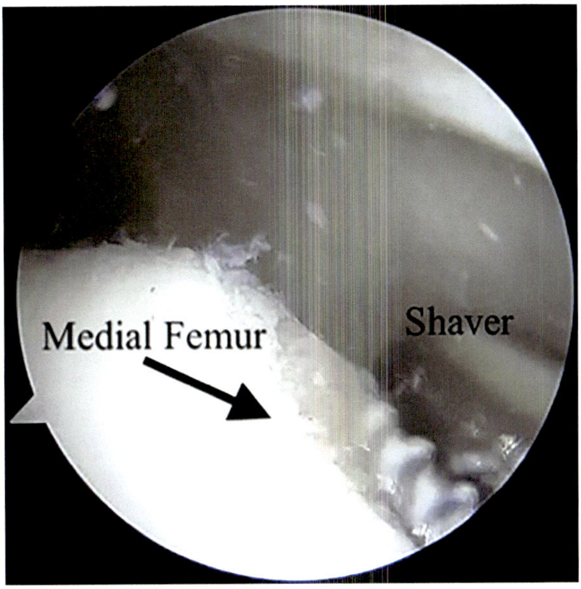

Fig. 5 The patient is supine with the right knee in full extension, we are viewing from the lateral portal with the 30° arthroscope. The shaver is shown obtaining medial femur non-articulating cartilage, with the GraftNet device applied to the shaver

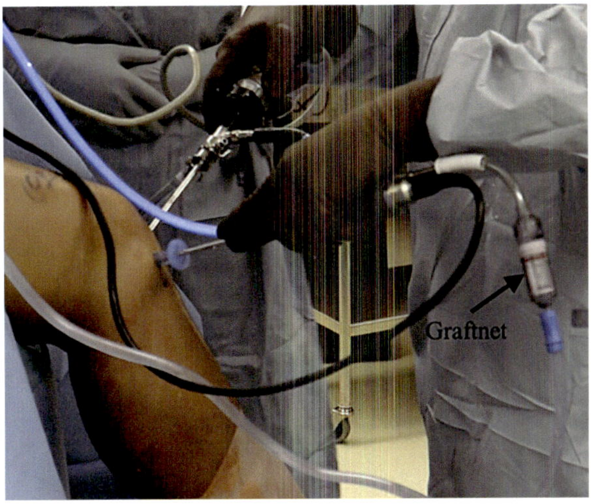

Fig. 6 With the right knee in 90% of flexion, the patient supine, and the 30° arthroscope placed through the medial portal, the shaver can be seen in the lateral portal, with the GraftNet device applied. The shaver harvests the lateral non-articulating cartilage

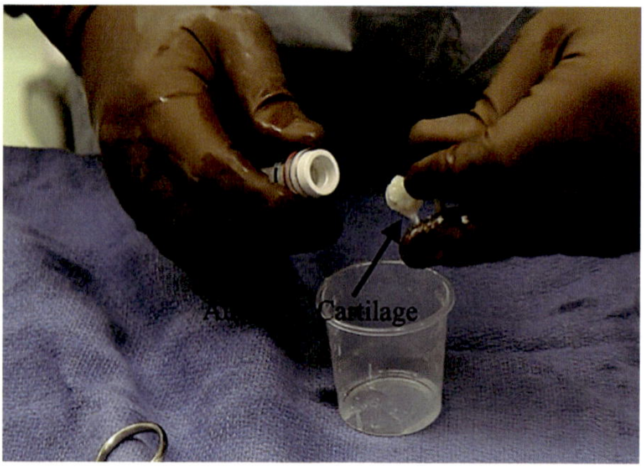

Fig. 7 The GraftNet device has been disassembled, and autograft cartilage is removed from the collector

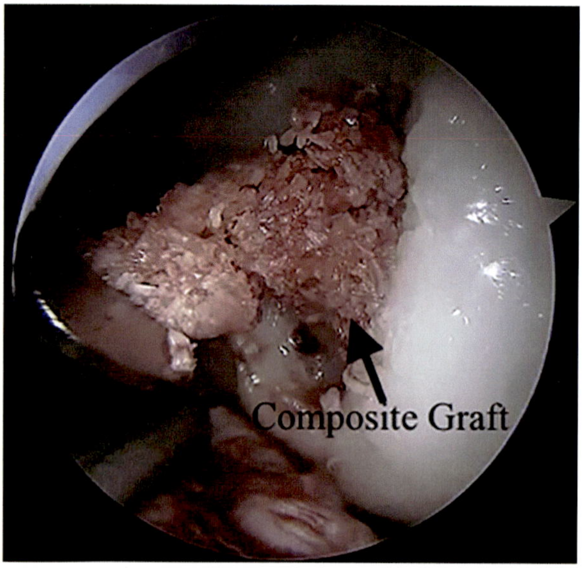

Fig. 8 With the patient supine, the right knee in 90% of flexion, and the 30° arthroscope placed through the medial portal, the composite graft is delivered through the lateral portal into the large osteochondral lesion on the lateral femoral condyle

non-articulating cartilage of the femur. This autograft cartilage is then carefully removed from the GraftNet device on the back table (Fig. 7).

After the harvesting process is complete, the composite graft is made. One milliliter of BioCartilage is added to the BioCartilage mixing cannula with the autograft cartilage. One milliliter of bone marrow concentrate is also added and mixed with the graft until a toothpaste consistency is obtained. The delivery cannula is then applied to the mixing cannula and placed on the back table.

During the graft delivery process, it may be helpful to establish an inferior accessory portal to aid in suctioning. The arthroscopy fluid is turned off at this point, and sponges can be used through the lateral portal to dry the lesion. The composite graft is then carefully delivered through the lateral portal, and a small bone tamp can be used to impact the graft in place (Figs. 8 and 9). The graft should not be prominent

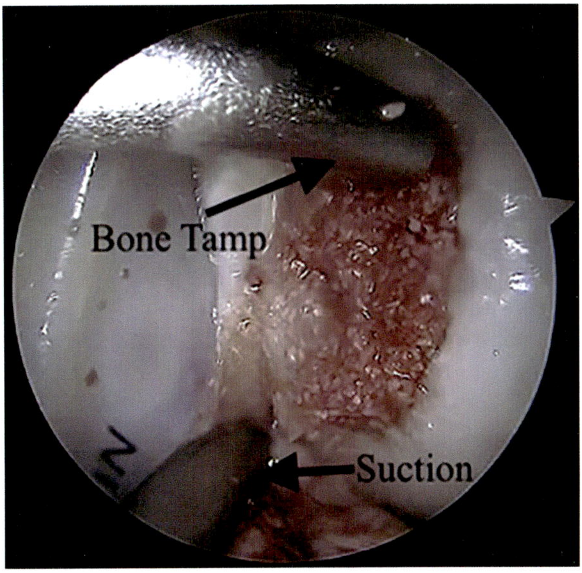

Fig. 9 With the patient supine, the right knee in 90% of flexion, and the arthroscope placed through the medial portal, a bone tamp has been placed through the lateral portal and is evening out the composite graft in the large osteochondral lesion on the lateral femoral condyle. A suction device has been placed through the inferior accessory portal

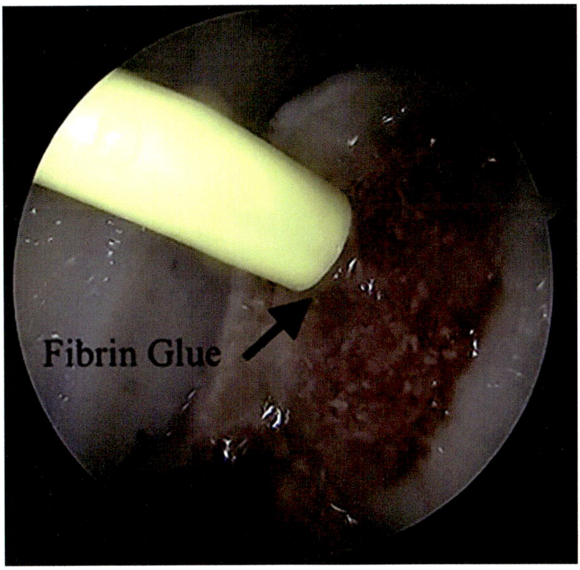

Fig. 10 With the patient supine, the right knee in 90% of flexion, and the arthroscope placed through the medial portal, a bone tamp has been placed through the lateral portal and is evening out the composite graft in the large osteochondral lesion on the lateral femoral condyle. A suction device has been placed through the inferior accessory portal

and should be contained within the defect. After the graft is properly placed into the lesion, Evicel glue (Ethicon, Blue Ash, OH) is delivered onto the graft. It is important to start the application of the glue superiorly because it will run inferiorly (Fig. 10). Care is taken not to deliver too much glue, and suction can be used to remove any excess. The glue will need at least 7–8 minutes to set up and fix the graft in place.

5 Discussion

Treatment of articular defects is difficult because of the avascular nature of hyaline cartilage. Most authors believe that treatment of osteochondral lesions should be based on skeletal maturity and lesion stability [5]. Osteochondral lesions in adults typically have an unremitting course and rarely respond to conservative measures. De Smet et al. reported only an 11% rate of good clinical outcomes in 9 knees after a mean follow-up period of 3.6 years [6]. Operative treatment should be considered in skeletally immature patients with detached or unstable lesions and those in which conservative measures have failed, as well as all lesions in adults, because the clinical course is deleterious, necessitating early aggressive intervention [4]. Drilling has been reported to be an effective technique in stable juvenile osteochondritis dissecans lesions. Aglietti et al. noted healing on radiographs after drilling in 16 knees in 14 patients, and all patients were asymptomatic at a mean follow-up of 4 years [7].

Unstable lesions should be treated operatively regardless of age. They should be further classified as salvageable or unsalvageable. Salvageable lesions are those with the potential for healing to the remainder of the subchondral bone with a congruent articular surface. Unsalvageable lesions are fragmented and cannot form a congruent articular surface with fixation because of excessive gapping. In cases of unsalvageable lesions and cases in which significant concern exists for the development of premature osteoarthritis, newer techniques have been developed to combat this problem. These include reparative techniques and restorative techniques. Reparative techniques such as microfracture and ACI aim to create fibrocartilaginous fill by addressing chondral lesions without subchondral bone loss. Restorative techniques such as osteochondral grafting allow for chondral as well as bony defects to be addressed.

Microfracture is used to create small perforations in subchondral bone, which release pluripotent cells from the marrow to create a fibrocartilage cap. ACI is a 2-stage procedure in which a small amount of hyaline cartilage is harvested arthroscopically and cultivated in the laboratory. The second stage of the procedure involves subsequent reimplantation of graft into the defect.

In an attempt to bypass the need for multiple procedures, as well as decrease donor-site morbidity, recent techniques have focused on single-stage procedures with transplantation of autologous hyaline cartilage fortified with bone marrow concentrate or plasma-rich protein. Buda et al. conducted a 1-step procedure in 20 patients with bone marrow-derived mesenchymal stem cells and platelet-rich fibrin [8]. The results of immunohistochemical analysis of biopsy specimens obtained from 2 patients showed type II cartilage, and MRI showed satisfactory filling of the articular defects. Cugat et al. presented 2 cases of patients treated with autologous mixed platelet-rich plasma and platelet-poor plasma with hyaline chips and intra-articular injection of platelet-rich plasma [9]. They noted a return to the preinjury level of play in both patients, with excellent defect filling on MRI (both patients) and arthroscopy (1 patient). Salzmann et al. presented a single-step surgical technique of autologous minced cartilage implantation with fibrin glue [10]. However, an open arthrotomy was used in this technique.

In this technique which is based on the article from Lavender et al. we perform a single-stage arthroscopic autologous chondrocyte transplantation using the GraftNet tissue collector [11]. Advantages of this technique include the minimally invasive nature and the fact that it is performed in a single stage. A disadvantage is that there are limited data on the viability of the cartilage cells obtained with the GraftNet device and their incorporation. Moreover, an obvious risk or disadvantage is that donor-site morbidity, although decreased, is still present. This technique circumvents the major drawbacks of previous techniques; however, further studies with long-term follow-up are needed to assess the effectiveness of the procedure.

6 Editor's View

During the creation of this technique, our goals were to attempt to utilize the most innovative and up-to-date biologic possibilities to create a procedure that was similar to the gold standard of an ACI. Through the use of the GraftNet and the BMC, we were able to take a technique which was biocartilage and even further enhance the autograft capabilities. This should lead to improved results in the future because as we know the gold standard is autologous cells. It should be noted that during the procedure we did take pathology of the cellular cartilage harvest which did show viable chondrocytes (Fig. 11). As you will see and have seen throughout the book this is just another way to utilize the GraftNet to obtain and utilize autograft cellular architecture in our reconstructions. I personally use this technique now where I was using BioCartilage alone or just microfracture and I look forward to seeing the results of this technique in the future. My hope is that the autograft cells that we are transferring are going to incorporate more of a native cartilage than what we have been able to obtain in the past with previous techniques.

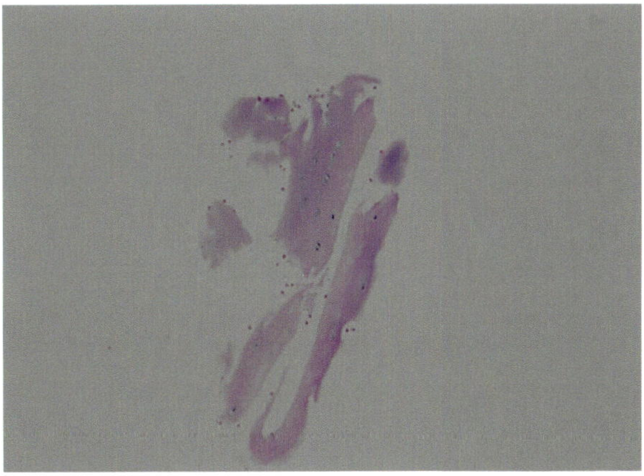

Fig. 11 Pathology image of cartilage which was harvested with the GraftNet

References

1. Detterline AJ, Goldstein JL, Rue JP, Bach BR Jr. Evaluation and treatment of osteochondritis dissecans lesions of the knee. J. Knee Surg. 2008;21:106–15.
2. Grimm NL, Weiss JM, Kessler JI, Aoki SK. Osteochondritis dissecans of the knee. Clin Sports Med. 2014;33:181–8.
3. Engasser W, Camp CL, Stuart MJ, Krych AJ. Current concepts in the treatment of osteochondral lesions of the knee. Minerva Ortop Traumatol. 2015;64:459–71.
4. Kocher MS, Tucker R, Ganley TJ, Flynn JM. Management of osteochondritis dissecans of the knee: current concepts review. Am. J. Sports Med. 2006;34:1181–91.
5. Edmonds EW, Polousky J. A review of knowledge in osteochondritis dissecans: 123 years of minimal evolution from König to the ROCK study group. Clin. Orthop. Relat. Res. 2013;471:1118–26.
6. De Smet AA, Ilahi OA, Graf BK. Untreated osteochondritis dissecans of the femoral condyles: prediction of patient outcome using radiographic and MR findings. Skelet. Radiol. 1997;26:463–7.
7. Aglietti P, Buzzi R, Bassi PB, Fioriti M. Arthroscopic drilling in juvenile osteochondritis dissecans of the medial femoral condyle. Arthroscopy. 1994;10:286–91.
8. Buda R, Vannini F, Cavallo M, Grigolo B, Cenacchi A, Giannini S. Osteochondral lesions of the knee: a new one-step repair technique with bone-marrow-derived cells. J. Bone Joint Surg. Am. 2010;92(suppl 2):2–11.
9. Cugat R, Alentorn-Geli E, Steinbacher G, et al. Treatment of knee osteochondral lesions using a novel clot of autologous plasma rich in growth factors mixed with healthy hyaline cartilage chips and intra-articular injection of PRGF. Case Rep. Orthop. 2017;2017:8284548.
10. Salzmann GM, Calek AK, Preiss S. Second-generation autologous minced cartilage repair technique. Arthrosc. Tech. 2017;6:e127–31.
11. Lavender C, Adil S, et al. Autograft cartilage transfer augmented with bone marrow concentrate and allograft cartilage extracellular matrix. Arthrosc Tech. 2020;9:e199–203.

Intraosseous Bioplasty of the Lateral Femoral Condyle of the Knee for Osteonecrosis

Jeeshan A. Faridi and Paul E. Caldwell

1 Introduction

The subchondral bone plays a critical biomechanical role in knee homeostasis by providing structural support to the overlying articular cartilage. The presence of altered joint mechanics may cause both acute and chronic areas of increased focal stress and subsequent bone marrow edema (BME). Additional causes of BME may be acute or repetitive trauma, insufficiency fractures, osteoarthritis, and osteonecrosis. The pathophysiology of BME has been well-described, and the increased intraosseous pressure (IOP) results in subsequent decreased perfusion of subchondral bone [1]. The limited blood supply in these regions compromises the ability to heal. The subchondral ischemia coupled with increased focal stress results in high bone turnover and abnormal remodeling with subsequent attritional bone loss.

Osteonecrosis may be challenging to diagnose since standard knee radiographs often fail to demonstrate any signs of the subchondral bone pathology in the early stages (Fig. 1). In more advanced cases, subchondral sclerosis and collapse, along with joint space narrowing are more recognizable findings. Once the disease has progressed to the late stages, only osteochondral and arthroplasty reconstructive treatment options remain. Optimal treatment of osteonecrosis requires early recognition to allow for potential biologic restoration. Magnetic resonance imaging (MRI) is excellent for detecting the increased water content associated with marrow edema and is subsequently the imaging modality of choice for timely detection and detailed evaluation of osteonecrosis.

J. A. Faridi
Orthopaedic Research of Virginia Sports Medicine Fellowship Program, Richmond, VA, USA

P. E. Caldwell (✉)
Orthopaedic Research of Virginia and Tuckahoe Orthopaedic Associates, Ltd., Richmond, VA, USA

C. Lavender (ed.), *Biologic and Nanoarthroscopic Approaches in Sports Medicine*, https://doi.org/10.1007/978-3-030-71323-2_7

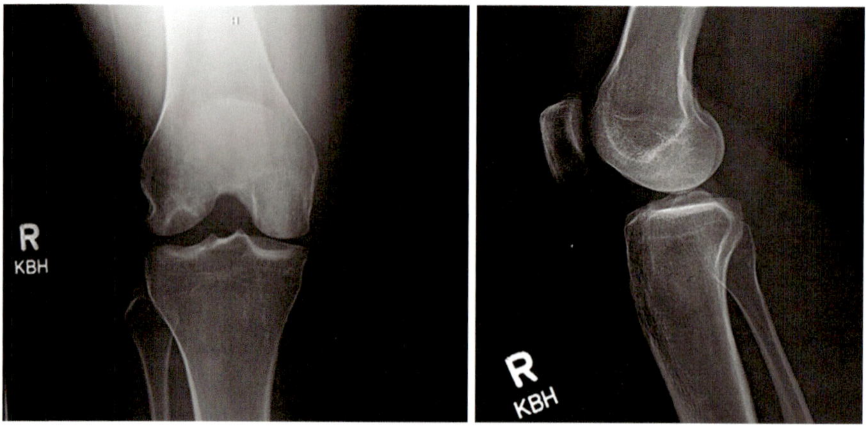

Fig. 1 AP and lateral radiograph of right knee demonstrating lytic lesion in lateral femoral condyle in a patient with secondary osteonecrosis

Patients with focal subchondral osteonecrotic lesions, without disruption of the articular cartilage or subchondral collapse, may be candidates for intraosseous bioplasty. The goal of this minimally invasive biologic treatment is to address the subchondral bone defects by reducing IOP, returning blood supply, and promoting bone remodeling. This technique utilizes fluoroscopic guidance to target the bone marrow lesion seen on MRI. Decompression of the lesion is followed by the injection of a combination of bone marrow aspirate concentrate (BMAC) and either autologous bone graft or allograft such as a demineralized bone matrix. This mixture delivers the osteoinductive, osteoconductive, and osteogenic factors necessary to promote bone healing and remodeling in an effort to diminish the patient's symptoms.

2 Indications/Contraindications

Bioplasty of the knee may be indicated for the treatment of numerous disorders of the knee, but the common finding in this diverse group of pathologies is BME. Although our description focuses on osteonecrosis of the knee, the intraosseous bioplasty technique may be applicable to other disorders of the knee that cause BME and the associated symptoms. The goal of this biologic treatment is to reduce symptoms of pain and ideally return patients to previous levels of function and allow them to lead an active lifestyle. This is especially important in younger, more active patients who wish to postpone joint arthroplasty.

Osteonecrosis of the knee was first described by Ahlback et al. in 1968 and can be a rapidly progressing disease that leads to end-stage arthritis [2]. The knee is the most common joint affected after the hip. Osteonecrosis of the knee is generally categorized into three types: primary or spontaneous osteonecrosis of the knee

(SONK), secondary (atraumatic, ischemic, or idiopathic osteonecrosis), and post-arthroscopic.

SONK is the most common form of osteonecrosis with the majority of patients being above 60 years of age. It is most often unilateral and affects women more than men. The prevalence is thought to be underestimated as many patients with end-stage osteoarthritis may have had undiagnosed SONK. It is believed to result from subchondral insufficiency fractures in osteopenic bone, leading to fluid accumulation, focal ischemia, and subsequent necrosis. The medial femoral condyle is most often affected due to the diminished extraosseous and intraosseous blood supply compared to the lateral femoral condyle [3].

Secondary osteonecrosis usually involves both condyles of the femur, and the opposite knee is involved 80% of the time [4]. Approximately 90% of cases are associated with alcohol abuse and corticosteroid use [5]. The pathophysiology is believed to be an increase in adipocyte size and number within the bone, leading to the displacement of the bone marrow. This increased pressure leads to vascular collapse and resultant ischemia [6]. The severity of osteonecrosis has been classified, and radiographs of Ficat stage I and II will have a normal joint space with no evidence of subchondral collapse. Stage II will show sclerosis in the trabeculae of the subchondral region. Stage III demonstrates a slightly narrowed joint space with some collapse of the subchondral bone and a crescent sign. Stage IV has a more significant joint-space narrowing, subchondral collapse, and further secondary degenerative changes [7] (Fig. 2). MRI is used to evaluate the progression of osteonecrosis and often demonstrates serpentine lesions with a well-demarcated border along with multiple foci of marrow involvement with extension into the metaphysis and diaphysis.

The reported incidence of post-arthroscopic osteonecrosis was found to be 4% by Cetik et al. with the medial femoral condyle comprising 82% of cases [8]. It has been proposed by Pape and colleagues that meniscectomized knee compartments undergo altered biomechanics and hoop stresses causing increased focal contact pressures which lead to insufficiency fractures with eventual necrosis [9].

Nonoperative treatment consists of medications, intra-articular injections, physical therapy, unloader braces, and activity modifications. Numerous surgical procedures have been proposed for patients that fail to improve after a trial of non-operative

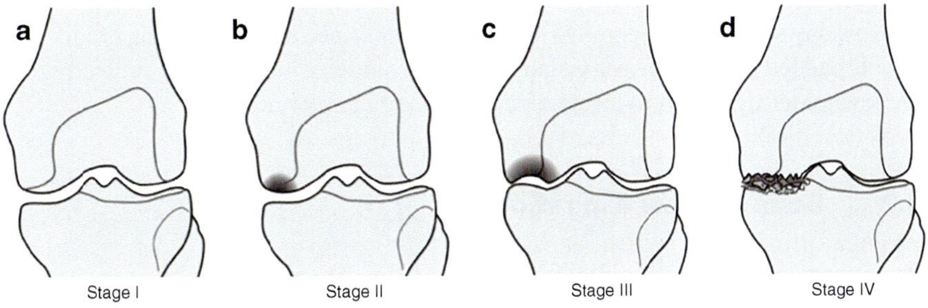

Fig. 2 (**a**–**d**) Ficat staging of osteonecrosis of the knee [7]

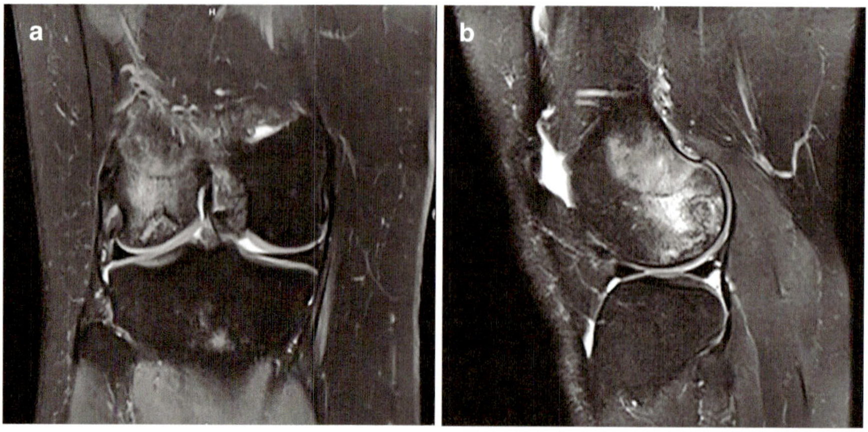

Fig. 3 Coronal (**a**) and sagittal (**b**) T2 fat-suppressed MRI image of the right knee demonstrating subchondral lesion with surrounding bone marrow edema in the lateral femoral condyle. As a result of increased water content, bone marrow edema on MRI demonstrates a hyperintense marrow signal on fluid sensitive, fat-suppressed sequences

treatment. Patients with radiographs and an MRI that demonstrate a focal lesion of subchondral BME without collapse are excellent candidates for intraosseous bioplasty (Fig. 3). This minimally invasive technique allows for concomitant arthroscopy to address intra-articular pathology such as meniscal tears or loose bodies. While a high tibial osteotomy alone has been advocated in the past to unload the affected condyle, bioplasty has the advantages of being a less-invasive and a less-morbid option. Patients with the collapse of the subchondral bone or cartilage loss are not indicated for bioplasty and may be more appropriate for osteochondral restoration or arthroplasty.

3 Technique

3.1 Positioning

The patient is positioned supine on the operating room table using the standard knee arthroscopy set-up. The operative leg is placed in a knee arthroscopy leg holder with a well-padded tourniquet proximally. The tourniquet is not initially inflated nor is the leg holder tightened to ensure adequate bone marrow aspirate.

3.2 Bone Marrow Aspiration

Bone marrow aspirate is initially harvested from the proximal tibia using a bone marrow trocar (Arthrex, Naples, FL). A stab incision is made just lateral to the tibial tubercle, and the trocar is advanced by hand approximately 3 cm past the cortex into

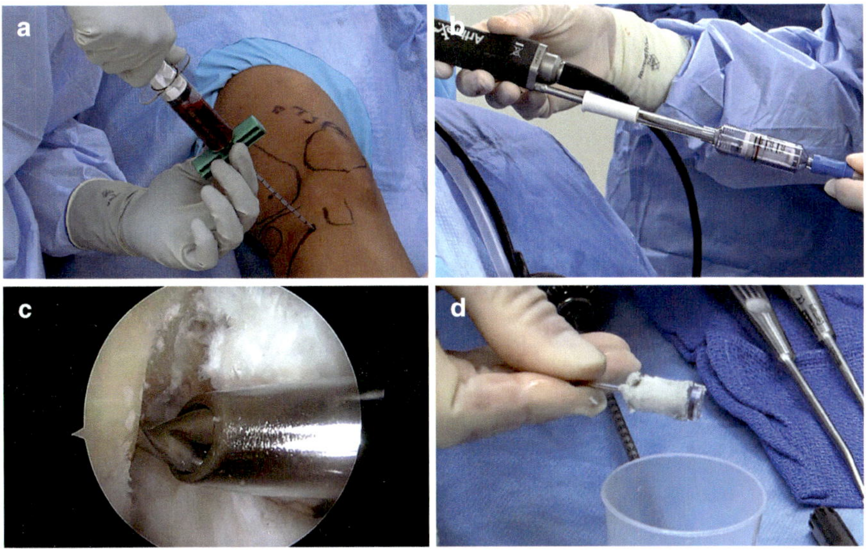

Fig. 4 (**a**) Bone marrow aspirate being obtained from the proximal tibia. (**b**) GraftNet autologous bone graft collection device attached to the arthroscopic shaver. (**c**) Arthroscopic image of bone being harvested from lateral femoral condyle. (**d**) Collected bone graft

the tibia. The trocar is calibrated so that distance from the cortex to the skin is recorded to ensure that the trocar is not advanced too deep. The stylus is removed, and a 30-cc syringe is secured on to the trocar and used to harvest the bone marrow aspirate. To aid in aspiration, the trocar may be periodically rotated 90° and slightly withdrawn to improve the harvest (Fig. 4a). The trocar may also be redirected through the same cortical hole to access additional bone marrow. Once the second syringe of bone marrow aspirate is obtained, the trocar is withdrawn and the aspirate is passed off the back table and prepared in the Angel bone marrow aspirate processing system (Arthrex).

3.3 Knee Arthroscopy and Bone Graft Harvest

Attention is then turned to arthroscopy of the knee. The leg is elevated and exsanguinated, the tourniquet is inflated, and the leg holder is tightened. A diagnostic arthroscopy is undertaken to evaluate the integrity of the articular cartilage covering the area of subchondral osteonecrosis as well as any concomitant pathology. Once the diagnostic portion of the arthroscopy has been completed and confirmation of healthy and stable cartilage is confirmed, attention is turned to the harvest of the autologous bone graft. Our preference is to harvest the bone graft arthroscopically from the lateral wall and roof of the notch of the knee using a burr (Arthrex) (Fig. 4c). The cartilage and soft tissue are removed from the harvest site, and care is taken to avoid iatrogenic injury to the insertion of the cruciate ligaments. Once the bone is exposed, the GraftNet (Arthrex) is applied to the shaver to collect the morselized bone (Fig. 4b). We would recommend harvesting approximately 3–4 cc of bone graft to be mixed with the BMAC. The bone graft is removed from the GraftNet and placed into the delivery and mixing syringe (Arthrex) to be combined with the BMAC (Fig. 4d). In the case of insufficient bone graft harvest, a demineralized bone matrix may be added to increase volume. The BMAC is combined with the bone graft to create a mixture consistent with "slush" (Fig. 5a). We prefer a ratio of 5 cc of bone graft to 4 cc of BMAC to ensure adequate viscosity for injection. One milliliter of radiopaque dye may be added to the mix to aid in fluoroscopic visualization and confirmation of adequate fill.

3.4 Bioplasty Technique

The region of subchondral osteonecrosis is customarily approached from the corresponding side of the femoral condyle using a percutaneous approach. The preoperative MRI is useful to have available in the operating room, but fluoroscopy is always used to confirm localization. A spinal needle is utilized to place the tip on the cortex to localize the subchondral osteonecrotic lesion under fluoroscopy. This is followed by a percutaneous incision and subsequent drilling of a 2.4-mm guidewire (Arthex) into the lesion (Fig. 5c). Once the placement of the guidewire is confirmed with fluoroscopy, a 7-mm cannulated reamer (Arthrex) is used to complete the core

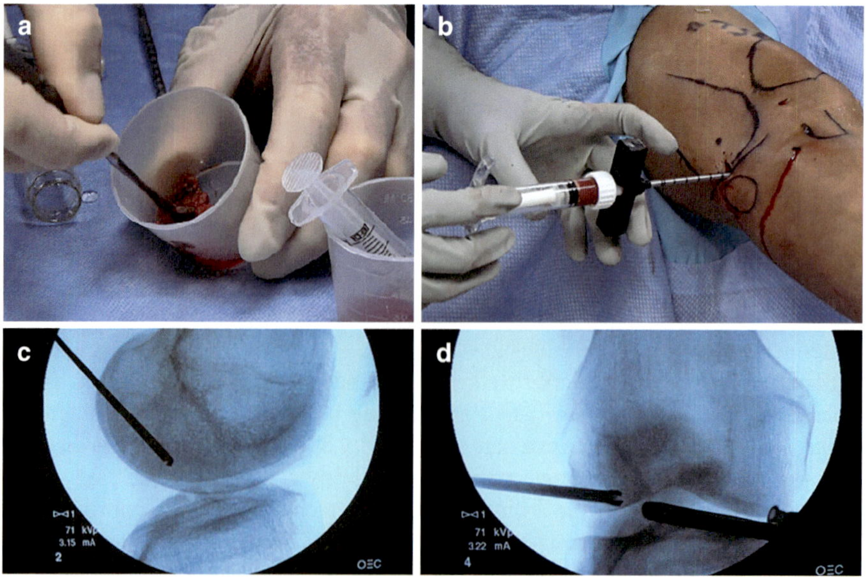

Fig. 5 (**a**) BMAC has been combined with bone autograft. (**b**) Biologic injection of BMAC and bone autograft placed in the lesion. Correct placement of injection is confirmed with the use of fluoroscopy (**c**, **d**)

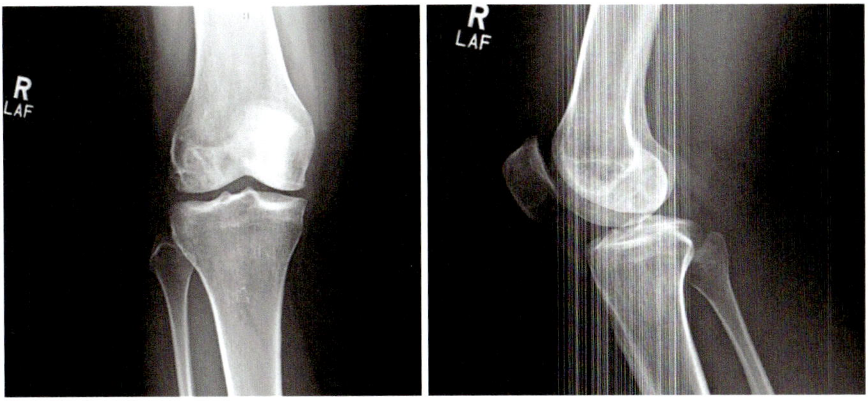

Fig. 6 AP and lateral radiograph of right knee demonstrating lesion in lateral femoral condyle approximately 4 months after bioplasty procedure for secondary osteonecrosis

decompression (Fig. 5d). Although fluoroscopic verification is essential, we recommend arthroscopic visualization of the cartilage surface during core decompression to ensure that the reamer does not violate the articular cartilage. The reamer is removed from the knee, leaving the guidewire in place. The inner style of the delivery cannula is removed, and the cannula is advanced over the guidewire. Once the delivery cannula position is confirmed under fluoroscopy, the guide wire is removed, and the mixing syringe is placed on to the back of the trocar (Fig. 5b). During injection, the trocar is slowly removed to ensure a complete fill of the core decompression void. Figure 6 demonstrates radiographs of the same lateral femoral condyle lesion as seen in Fig. 1 approximately 4 months after the bioplasty procedure.

We endorse the addition of radiopaque dye into the mixture to aid in fluoroscopic confirmation. If notable resistance is encountered with attempted injection, the BioXpress cannula (Arthrex) may be used to decrease resistance as it has a larger delivery diameter.

4 Discussion

Osteonecrosis of the hip in the young patient has been well studied, and current recommendations are for early diagnosis and treatment to avoid the catastrophic consequence of collapse of the articular cartilage and subsequent need for arthroplasty [10]. Similar to the hip, osteonecrosis of the knee is now more commonly recognized as a source of pain and disability. The pathophysiology is thought to be due to a decreased blood supply to the subchondral region of the bone and subsequent microfracture of trabecular bone. It is well documented that both the activity and number of mesenchymal stem cells in the hematopoietic and stromal compartments of the bone marrow are decreased in patients with osteonecrosis [10].

Historically, the gold standard surgical procedure for early-stage osteonecrosis of the femoral head was core decompression. More recently, core decompression has been combined with injection of autologous bone marrow cells with good results [11, 12]. At a 5-year follow-up, 8 of 11 patients treated with decompression only went on to hip replacement compared to only 3 out of 13 treated with decompression and injection of bone marrow cells [13]. A randomized controlled trial performed by Ma et al. in 2014 demonstrated no progression of osteonecrosis in 100% of Ficat stage 1 and 2 patients in the treatment group and 66% in the control group treated without bone marrow cell implantation at 2-year follow-up [14]. Successful outcomes for the treatment of osteonecrosis in the hip have influenced the evolution of the development of the intraosseous bioplasty technique for the treatment of bone marrow lesions in the knee.

Core decompression for the treatment of osteonecrosis in the knee was first described in 1989 by Jacobs et al. They performed 28 core decompressions of the distal femur for avascular necrosis over a 7-year period and had a mean follow-up of 54 months. All 7 patients with Ficat stages I and II had good results. Of the 21 patients in stage III, 11 cases had good results, 4 had poor results, and 6 progressed to total knee replacement [15]. Even without the added benefit of BMAC and autograft bone, Marulanda et al. reported a 92% success rate with percutaneous decompression combined with limited weight-bearing for 4–6 weeks in secondary osteonecrosis [16]. Mont et al. presented their results of core decompression compared to protected weight bearing in 79 knees with osteonecrosis due to corticosteroid use. A subset of 26 knees from each group was matched for age, gender, diagnosis, Ficat and Arlet Stage, and length of follow-up. The matched protected weight-bearing group had 23% survival as compared with 74% survival in the core decompression group, and they concluded that surgical treatment may slow the rate of symptomatic progression of avascular necrosis of the knee and delay the need for more extensive procedures such as total knee arthroplasty [17].

Bone marrow edema in the knee has been strongly associated with pain, decreased function, cartilage damage, and progression to knee replacement [18, 19]. Previous studies have determined that IOP is approximately 97% higher in patients with BME versus those without and that increased IOP is associated with an increase in knee pain [20, 21]. In 2019, Kasik et al. initially published a case series of patients undergoing bioplasty in the knee for bone marrow edema [22]. They demonstrated statistically significant improvement in both visual analog scale (VAS) and International Knee Documentation Committee (IKDC) scores in 19 of 20 patients. They reported on 14 patients at 1-year follow-up, and only 1 required an arthroplasty procedure. Although all of these patients had concomitant pathology addressed at the time of the procedure (partial medial meniscectomy [70%], chondroplasty [25%], and partial lateral meniscectomy [20%]), short-term results are encouraging. Bioplasty has also been described in the treatment of subchondral cysts in both the lateral femoral condyle and lateral tibial plateau [23, 24]. Its use is also being studied in the capitellum, talus, patella, and proximal humerus. Additional long-term studies are necessary to provide affirmation of the efficacy of intraosseous bioplasty in the knee for the treatment of bone marrow lesions.

Utilizing intraosseous bioplasty in the treatment of focal subchondral osteonecrotic lesions of the knee has a distinct set of advantages over previously described more invasive techniques utilizing an arthrotomy or osteotomy. The entire procedure is performed through arthroscopic portals and percutaneous incisions. The bone marrow is aspirated from the proximal tibia, simplifying both prepping and draping, without the need to access the iliac crest. The use of BMAC provides osteoinductive factors and osteogenic stem cells, which are not found with simple decompression procedures. The ability to harvest the autologous bone graft arthroscopically using the burr and GraftNet is less invasive and morselizes the bone graft which allows easy delivery without the need for manual compression. Delivery of an osteoconductive scaffold along with osteoinductive factors into the previously decompressed lesion provides potential for more rapid incorporation compared to allograft or demineralized bone matrix.

Arthroscopic autograft harvest from the lateral femoral condyle has some distinct disadvantages. Graft harvest morbidity is always a concern, although our technique minimizes this risk by avoiding violation of the articular cartilage. The limited amount of graft that can be harvested arthroscopically may be problematic depending on the size of the lesion. We recommend augmentation with a demineralized bone matrix if the need arises. Special care should be taken to avoid iatrogenic damage to the cruciate ligament insertions during harvest and intermittently probing to monitor is recommended. Cost is also a concern, and the use of both the Arthrex GraftNet and Angel systems, in addition to the possible allograft, may be cost-prohibitive in an outpatient setting.

5 Editor's View

AVN and bone marrow lesions are difficult issues to treat because of poor biology. In this technique, we counteract that biology with the addition of the latest orthobiologics available. It is a straightforward technique for harvesting and delivery. It is a great option now to add in autograft tissue as seen here to perform the bioplasty in the hope we improve outcomes for this condition.

References

1. Kiaer T, Dahl B, Lausten GS. The relationship between inert gas wash-out and radioactive tracer microspheres in measurement of bone blood flow: effect of decreased arterial supply and venous congestion on bone blood flow in an animal model: Inert gas wash-out and bone blood flow. J Orthop Res. 1993;11:28–35.
2. Ahlbäck S, Bauer GC, Bohne WH. Spontaneous osteonecrosis of the knee. Arthritis Rheum. 1968;11:705–33.
3. Reddy AS, Frederick RW. Evaluation of the intraosseous and extraosseous blood supply to the distal femoral condyles. Am J Sports Med. 1998;26(3):415–9.
4. Mont MA, Marker DR, Zywiel MG, et al. Osteonecrosis of the knee and related conditions. J Am Acad Orthop Surg. 2011;19:482–94.

5. Mont MA, Baumgarten KM, Rifai A, et al. Atraumatic osteonecrosis of the knee. J Bone Joint Surg Am. 2000;82:1279–90.
6. Lerebours F, ElAttrache NS, Mandelbaum B. Diseases of subchondral bone 2. Sports Med Arthrosc Rev. 2016;24(2):50–5.
7. Michael K-O, Kody B, Monti K. Algorithm for treatment of hip and knee osteonecrosis: review and a presentation of three example cases. J Rheum Dis Treat. 2017;3(3):053.
8. Cetik O, Cift H, Comert B, et al. Risk of osteonecrosis of the femoral condyle after arthroscopic chondroplasty using radiofrequency: a prospective clinical series. Knee Surg Sports Traumatol Arthrosc. 2009;17:24–9.
9. Pape D, Seil R, Anagnostakos K, et al. Postarthroscopic osteonecrosis of the knee. Arthroscopy. 2007;23:428–38.
10. Hernigou P, Beaujean F, Lambotte JC. Decrease in the mesenchymal stem cell pool in the proximal femur in corticosteroid-induced osteonecrosis. J Bone Joint Surg (Br). 1999;81:349–55.
11. Hernigou P, Beaujean F. Treatment of osteonecrosis with autologous bone marrow grafting. Clin Orthop. 2002;405:14–23.
12. Hernigou P, Poignard A, Zilber S, et al. Cell therapy of hip osteonecrosis with autologous bone marrow grafting. Indian J Orthop. 2009;43:40–5.
13. Gangji V, De Maertelaer V, Hauzeur J-P. Autologous bone marrow cell implantation in the treatment of non-traumatic osteonecrosis of the femoral head: five year follow-up of a prospective controlled study. Bone. 2011;49(5):1005–9.
14. Ma Y, Wang T, Liao J, et al. Efficacy of autologous bone marrow buffy coat grafting combined with core decompression in patients with avascular necrosis of femoral head: a prospective, double-blinded, randomized, controlled study. Stem Cell Res Ther. 2014;5:115.
15. Jacobs MA, Loeb PE, Hungerford DS. Core decompression of the distal femur for avascular necrosis of the knee. J Bone Joint Surg (Br). 1989;71:583–7.
16. Marulanda G, Seyler TM, Sheikh NH, et al. Percutaneous drilling for the treatment of secondary osteonecrosis of the knee. J Bone Joint Surg (Br). 2006;88:740–6.
17. Mont MA, Tomek IM, Hungerford DS. Core decompression for avascular necrosis of the distal femur: long term followup. Clin Orthop Relat Res. 1997;334:124–30.
18. Tanamas SK, Wluka AE, Pelletier J-P, et al. Bone marrow lesions in people with knee osteoarthritis predict progression of disease and joint replacement: a longitudinal study. Rheumatology. 2010;49:2413–9.
19. Scher C, Craig J, Nelson F. Bone marrow edema in the knee in osteoarthrosis and association with total knee arthroplasty within a three-year follow-up. Skelet Radiol. 2008;37:609–17.
20. Uchio Y, Ochi M, Adachi N, Nishikori T, Kawasaki K. Intraosseous hypertension and venous congestion in osteonecrosis of the knee. Clin Orthop. 2001;384:217–23.
21. Arnoldi CC, Lemperg K, Linderholm H. Intraosseous hypertension and pain in the knee. J Bone Joint Surg (Br). 1975;57(3):360–3.
22. Kasik CS, Martinkovich S, Mosier B, Akhavan S. Short-term outcomes for the biologic treatment of bone marrow edema of the knee using bone marrow aspirate concentrate and injectable demineralized bone matrix. Arthrosc Sports Med Rehabil. 2019;1(1):e7–e14.
23. Elena N, Woodall BM, Lee K, et al. Intraosseous bioplasty for a chondral cyst in the lateral tibial plateau. Arthrosc Tech. 2018;7(11):e1149–56.
24. Potty AGR, Gupta A, Rodriguez HC, Stone IW, Maffulli N. Intraosseous bioplasty for a subchondral cyst in the lateral condyle of femur. J Clin Med. 2020;9(5):1358.

The Use of Cartiform in the Knee for Osteochondral Defects

Christopher Wang and Sam Akhavan

1 Introduction

Articular cartilage defects of the knee can occur as a spectrum in young, active patients. These range from focal, single defects to diffuse articular degeneration of cartilage. Injuries such as these pose a complicated problem for surgeons, especially when treating younger, active patients. The first described attempt at implantation of allograft cartilage was by Henri Judet [1], which was performed using animal models. The first documented human allograft cartilage transplants in a clinical setting did not occur until 1908 [1].

Historically, treatment of cartilage lesions has been performed using both mechanical and biological treatment options. Malalignment of the knee and/or ligament insufficiency are treated typically with some type of osteotomy procedure (high tibial osteotomy, distal femoral, or tibial tuberosity) and/or ligament reconstruction. If the patellofemoral joint is involved, then an anteromedialization procedure can be performed as well [2].

Once these have been addressed, then attention can be turned to the cartilage lesion itself. Microfracture involves drilling multiple holes into the subchondral bone, about 2–3 mm apart. This allows for a fibrin clot to be created, aiding in the transfer of stem cells and pluripotent cells to the injured area, resulting in a fibrocartilage "fill" of the defect [3, 4]. Osteochondral autograft transplantation is performed by transfer of a single or multiple cylindrical osteochondral plugs into the cartilage defect [5]. This can result in a hyaline-covered cartilage repair [4, 6]. Autologous chondrocyte implantation (ACI) and matrix-associated chondrocyte implantation (MACI) can be used for focal cartilage defects with minimal bone loss underneath

C. Wang (✉)
Allegheny Health Network, Pittsburgh, PA, USA
e-mail: Christopher.Wang@AHN.ORG

S. Akhavan
Orthopaedic Sports Medicine, Allegheny Health Network, Pittsburgh, PA, USA

C. Lavender (ed.), *Biologic and Nanoarthroscopic Approaches in Sports Medicine*, https://doi.org/10.1007/978-3-030-71323-2_8

[6]. These procedures involve harvesting native cartilage during an initial arthroscopic evaluation, then 6 weeks later implanting the harvested cartilage as a flap onto the defect [3].

Osteochondral allograft transplantation offers a treatment option for a wide range of cartilage injuries. It involves the transfer of cadaveric graft that includes both the hyaline cartilage surface and subchondral bone. Allografts are available as fresh, fresh-frozen, and cryo-preserved [7]. Fresh osteochondral allografts offer the highest concentration of viable chondrocytes; however, they have a much shorter shelf-life with recommendations of use within 28–30 days of harvest from the donor [8, 9]. Due to the need for bacterial and viral testing prior to implantation, these grafts often have only a 2-week window during which to be used and implanted.

Fresh-frozen and cryopreserved allografts have the significant advantage of a much longer shelf life, but have a lower concentration of viable chondrocytes [9]. Cartiform® is a cryopreserved, osteochondral allograft currently produced by Arthrex (Naples, FL). The purpose of this chapter is to discuss the indications, contraindications, and technical guidelines in utilizing Cartiform® for cartilage defects in the knee.

2 Indications/Contraindications

Indications for any cartilage restoration procedures typically fall into two categories: lesion size and activity level of the patient. Table 1 provides a general algorithm for the treatment of cartilage defects depending on location in the knee as well as the aforementioned categories. Any cartilage lesions measuring less than 4 cm^2 or concomitant areas of bone loss can be treated with Cartiform®. The procedure can be done for both first-line or second-line treatment of lesions in the knee.

Relative contraindications include a large defect size measuring larger than 5 cm^2, given that the largest graft size available is 2 × 2.5 cm. Larger injury zones could be performed using Cartiform® but would require multiple grafts to be used. Large bony defects would also be considered a relative contraindication. As the grafts have only a thin layer of bone, either bone graft has to be used in conjunction for large bony defects or placing an osteochondral allograft plug instead. While the grafts are extensively tested, there is a theoretical risk of disease transmission that is related to any type of allograft substitute.

Table 1 General surgical algorithm for cartilage defects of the knee

Femoral condyle defect	Patellofemoral defect
<4 cm^2: microfracture, osteochondral autograft transfer <5 cm^2: Cartiform®	<4 cm^2: microfracture, osteochondral autograft transfer <5 cm^2: Cartiform®
>4 cm^2: osteochondral allograft transplantation, autologous chondrocyte implantation	>4 cm^2: autologous chondrocyte implantation, microfracture for low demand/elderly patients

3 Surgical Technique

3.1 Preoperative Preparation and Patient Positioning

The patient is placed in a supine position on a regular table. Preoperative antibiotics are given. A lateral post is placed on the operative extremity side as it will be used for the arthroscopic evaluation portion of the procedure. The leg is then prepped and draped in the typical fashion.

3.2 Arthroscopic Evaluation

A standard anterolateral portal is placed first for scope placement. A diagnostic exam is then performed to evaluate the other compartments of the knee. An anteromedial portal is placed under direct visualization. A probe is then placed through this portal to evaluate the area of the cartilage lesion (Fig. 1). Any loose cartilage debris should be debrided in order to clearly define the size of the lesion. The lesion is measured utilizing the tip of the probe and checked against the measurement done on the MRI. Once satisfied with the measurements, the instruments and scope are removed. Any lesion measuring 5 cm^2 or less would be a good candidate for a Cartiform®.

Tips and Pearls A determination of the appropriate size and shape of the defect is key to success prior to arthrotomy. The Cartiform® is available in 1 cm^2 disc, 2 cm^2

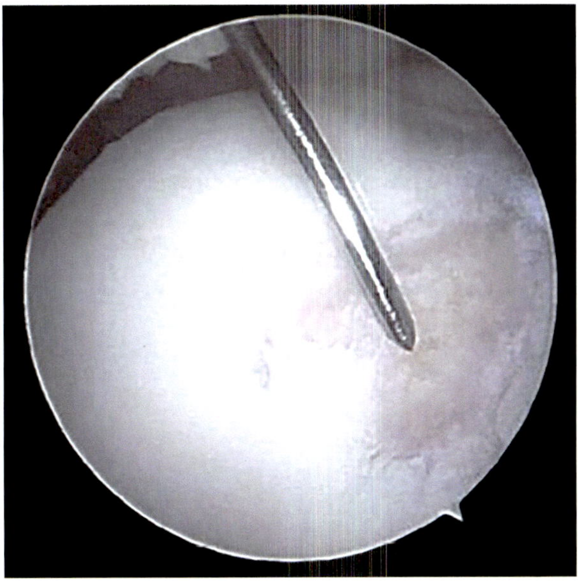

Fig. 1 The cartilage lesion is identified and debrided to show the extent of the defect. In this case, the defect was along the trochlear groove

disc, and 2 × 2.5 cm^2. The size of the defect can often be underestimated unless all loose cartilage is removed.

3.3 Cartilage Site Preparation

Depending on the location of the lesion, either a formal medial or lateral arthrotomy is made with an incision 6- to 8-cm in length. Once the patella is able to be mobilized, it is retracted out of the surgical field. Once the area of the diseased cartilage is identified, the area is debrided with curettes and shavers. This is taken down to bleeding, subchondral bone (Fig. 2). The borders of the lesion are sharply lined out with curettes or a scalpel until normal cartilage is seen. It is important to create stable margins for graft placement. Once fully visualized and cleaned, either a probe or ruler is used to measure out the diameter of the area to allow for correct sizing of the graft. The size of the defect can be mapped using paper or tin foil from either gloves or sterile suture packaging. The surgeon may or may not microfracture the area prior to placement of the graft.

Tips and Pearls The bony layer on the undersurface of the graft provides a healing surface to the defect. Make sure to get down to a good bleeding bone surface.

3.4 Graft Preparation

The Cartiform®(Arthrex) graft is a cryopreserved, osteochondral allograft that has intact cartilage with a thin layer of bone attached. The surface is perforated to allow flexibility to aid in handling and placement of the graft. The graft comes in a sterile jar and should be transferred onto the field into a sterile basin. Sterile saline is then added into the basin until just below the lid. This is allowed to thaw for a minimum of 10 minutes until no ice crystals are visible. The graft may then be taken out with sterile forceps and placed into sterile saline for at least 1 minute. It can remain in sterile saline for up to 2 hours at room temperature before implantation. There is a score mark on the graft that indicates the bottom side for placement.

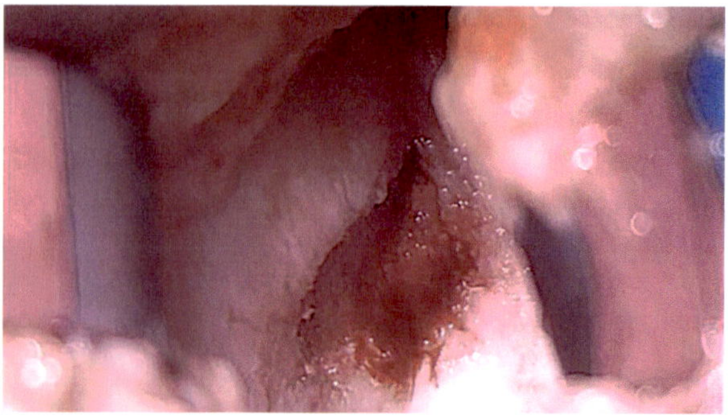

Fig. 2 A formal arthrotomy is performed into the knee. The cartilage lesion is fully debrided to bleeding bone and the edges cleaned

3.5 Graft Placement

The allograft can be cut to size with either Metzenbaum scissors or a scalpel. A pilot hole is placed in the center of the defect and a Knotless SutureTak® (Arthrex, Inc, Naples, FL) is implanted. Pilot holes may be placed along the periphery of the defect for PushLock® anchors before or after the initial placement of the graft. The central anchor suture is placed from the posterior aspect of the graft anteriorly, then back posteriorly to create a mattress stitch in the center. The tail is then placed through the FiberLink™ shuttling suture to fixate the strand into the anchor. The suture tail is then carried back from posterior to anterior direction in the center of the graft. This allows tension to be pulled directly on top of the graft. Again, the bottom (bone) side of the allograft has a score mark, and this should be placed onto the subchondral bone side. If the PushLock® anchors have not been placed yet, then at this point they can be drilled along the periphery of the lesion. Mattress sutures are placed along the edge of the graft and placed into those anchor points to achieve knotless fixation (Figs. 3, 4, and 5). A thin layer of fibrin glue may be placed along the periphery of the graft if desired.

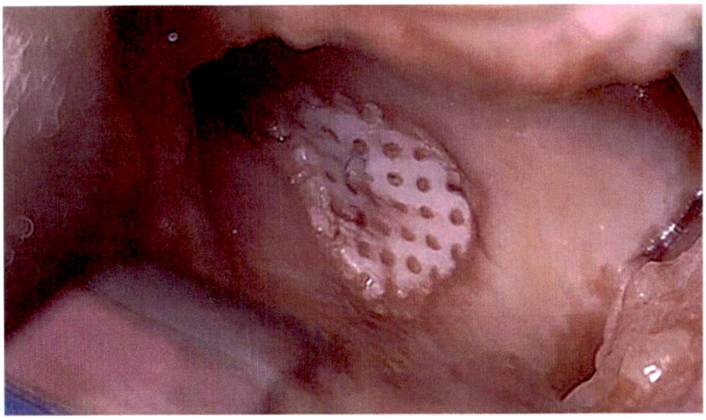

Fig. 3 The graft has been placed into the defect with a knotless suturetak placed in the center and four pushlock anchors along the periphery. No fibrin glue was used in this case

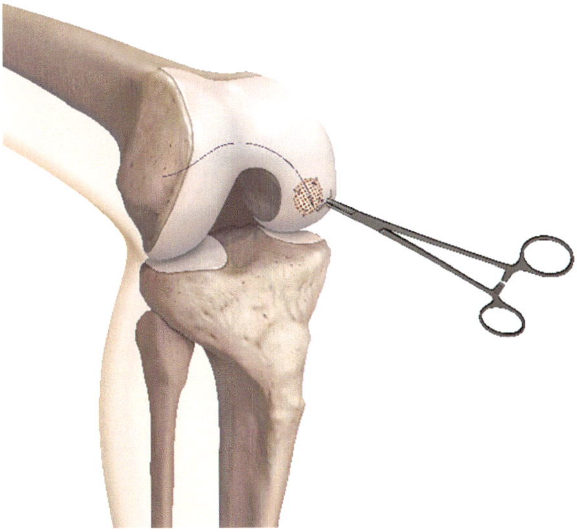

Fig. 4 Mattress sutures being placed into the graft. (Courtesy of Arthrex Inc. Naples, FL)

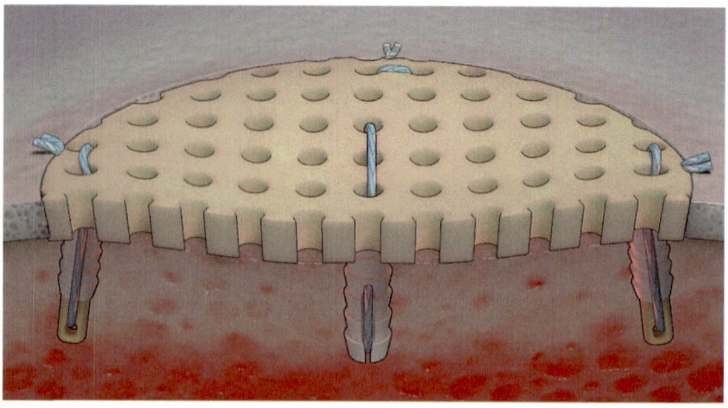

Fig. 5 Image of the final construct. (Courtesy of Arthrex Inc. Naples, FL)

Tips and Pearls The graft is malleable to the size and shape of the defect. In concave defects, placing an anchor in the center of the defect will allow the graft to match the concavity. Extraneous prominent graft on the edge of the defect can be shaped using a scalpel or the arthroscopic shaver.

3.6 Postoperative Protocol

The operative extremity is placed into an IROM brace. This is locked in full extension with the patient remaining non-weight bearing for at least 4–6 weeks to allow graft integration. The brace is unlocked on a week-to-week basis to allow a gradual range of motion for rehabilitation. After this non-weight bearing period, the patient will gradually progress from partial to full-weight bearing with physical therapy.

4 Discussion

Cartilage injuries of the knee can be devastating, especially to the younger population. There are a wide range of procedures and indications for this pathology. Microfracture remains a steadfast procedure used for smaller lesions or lower demand patients [6]. Osteochondral autografts can be used for lesions that include subchondral bone loss [10]. Lesions that are only isolated to the cartilage surface and that are in younger patients may be treated with an autologous chondrocyte implantation (ACI) or the current generation matrix-associated autologous chondrocyte implantation (MACI) [10]. Osteochondral allograft transplantation offers flexibility when treating large lesions that may not be candidates for microfracture or are too large for autograft transplants.

Osteochondral allografts have multiple uses both in the knee and other major joints of the body. Chahla et al. [11] performed a systematic review of clinical outcomes and failure rates of allograft transplantation in the patellofemoral joint. Their review included both fresh and cryopreserved grafts. Five- and 10-year survival rates were high, and outcome scores increased from pre- to post-operative status. McCulloch et al. [12] provided a case series of 25 patients with allograft transplants in the femoral condyles. Prospective data was collected, and statistically significant improvement was seen for every patient. Radiographically, 88% of the grafts were incorporated into the bone after 2 years. Murphy et al. [13] had a case series of 39 patients younger than 18 years of age that underwent osteochondral allograft transplantation for various lesions in the knee. Although 5 knees underwent a revision osteochondral allograft surgery, there was a 90% graft survivorship at 10 years, highlighting its effectiveness even in the younger age group.

Cartiform® is a cryopreserved allograft that has a thin layer of bone to allow for bony integration. Geraghty et al. [14] showed that cryopreserved osteochondral allograft retains viable chondrocytes, chondrogenic factors, and extracellular matrix proteins within native intact hyaline cartilage. It can be used not only for femoral condyle lesions, but can cover lesions of the patellofemoral joint as well [15]. Mirzayan et al. [9] describe the use of Cartiform® in the glenohumeral joint. This helps show the versatility of the graft in multiple scenarios where cartilage defects may appear.

In conclusion, Cartiform® offers a novel way to treat cartilage lesions in both young and older populations. It has the flexibility and sizes to cover most medium-to-large lesions of the knee. Since it is an allograft, there is less morbidity to the patient and the procedure can be done in one setting. However, since it is an allograft, there is a small chance of disease transmission because it is a cadaveric graft. Also, the cost of the graft itself may limit the availability of its use in certain facilities. Despite this, the graft offers the surgeon another option when treating cartilage injuries in the knee.

5 Editor's View

I have found this technique to be extremely useful in my practice especially in settings where you want more substance than the standard Biocartilage or microfracture options. Cartiform offers both substance and biology which are keys to treating cartilage lesions. As described here, lesion size and characteristics decide whether to use Cartiform, Autograft Cartilage Transfer, or other larger techniques.

References

1. Nikolaou VS, Giannoudis PV. History of osteochondral allograft transplantation. Injury. https://doi.org/10.1016/j.injury.2017.05.005.
2. Bode G, Schmal H, Pestka JM, Ogon P, Südkamp NP, Niemeyer P. A non-randomized controlled clinical trial on autologous chondrocyte implantation (ACI) in cartilage defects of the medial femoral condyle with or without high tibial osteotomy in patients with varus deformity of less than 5°. Arch. Orthop. Trauma Surg. 2012;133(1):43–9. https://doi.org/10.1007/s00402-012-1637-x.
3. Cole BJ, et al. Surgical management of articular cartilage defects in the knee. J. Bone Joint Surg. 2009;91(7):1778–90.
4. Magnussen RA, et al. Treatment of focal articular cartilage defects in the knee. Clin. Orthop. Relat. Res. 2008;466(4):952–62. https://doi.org/10.1007/s11999-007-0097-z.

5. Alford JW, Cole BJ. Cartilage restoration, part 2: techniques, outcomes, and future directions. Am. J. Sports Med. 2005;33(3):443–60. https://doi.org/10.1177/0363546505274578.
6. Bedi A, et al. Management of articular cartilage defects of the knee. J Bone Joint Surg Am. 2010;92(4):994–1009. https://doi.org/10.2106/jbjs.i.00895.
7. Alford JW, Cole BJ. Cartilage restoration, part 1. Am. J. Sports Med. 2005;33(2):295–306. https://doi.org/10.1177/0363546504273510.
8. Cavendish PA, et al. Osteochondral allograft transplantation for knee cartilage and osteochondral defects. JBJS Rev. 2019;7(6) https://doi.org/10.2106/jbjs.rvw.18.00123.
9. Mirzayan R, et al. Cryopreserved, viable osteochondral allograft for the treatment of a full-thickness cartilage defect of the glenoid. Arthrosc. Tech. 2018;7(12) https://doi.org/10.1016/j.eats.2018.08.013.
10. Chahla J, Stone J, Mandelbaum BR. How to manage cartilage injuries? Arthroscopy. 2019;35(10):2771–3. https://doi.org/10.1016/j.arthro.2019.08.021.
11. Chahla J, et al. Osteochondral allograft transplantation in the patellofemoral joint: a systematic review. Am. J. Sports Med. 2018;47(12):3009–18. https://doi.org/10.1177/0363546518814236.
12. Mcculloch PC, et al. Prospective evaluation of prolonged fresh osteochondral allograft transplantation of the femoral condyle. Am. J. Sports Med. 2007;35(3):411–20. https://doi.org/10.1177/0363546506295178.
13. Murphy RT, et al. Osteochondral allograft transplantation of the knee in the pediatric and adolescent population. Am. J. Sports Med. 2014;42(3):635–40. https://doi.org/10.1177/0363546513516747.
14. Geraghty S, Kuang J, Yoo D, et al. A novel, cryopreserved, viable osteochondral allograft designed to augment marrow stimulation for articular cartilage repair. J. Orthop. Surg. Res. 2015;10:66. https://doi.org/10.1186/s13018-015-0209-5.
15. Woodmass JM, et al. Viable osteochondral allograft for the treatment of a full-thickness cartilage defect of the patella. Arthrosc. Tech. 2017;6(5) https://doi.org/10.1016/j.eats.2017.06.034.

Superior Capsular Reconstruction of the Shoulder

Andrew Wilhelm and Sam Akhavan

1 Introduction

Superior capsular reconstruction (SCR) has become an increasingly popular technique for irreparable rotator cuff tears since Mihata first introduced his concept of the procedure in 2012 [1]. SCR is indicated for an irreparable or previously failed rotator cuff repair with poor tissue quality, in the setting of minimal to no glenohumeral arthritis. This difficult clinical scenario has been traditionally treated in a multitude of ways, none of which have provided sustained results similar to a primary rotator cuff repair [2]. When an elderly patient presents with an irreparable rotator cuff tear, the surgical option of a reverse total shoulder arthroplasty may very well be a viable and reliable option; however, in the face of a younger patient with higher functional demands and expectations, this surgical option is less than ideal.

Non-operative treatments for irreparable rotator cuff tears including physical therapy have had far inferior results to surgical counterparts; thus, this condition is typically treated surgically [3]. Surgical options used to treat an irreparable rotator cuff repair have included debridement with subacromial decompression, partial rotator cuff repair, muscle transfers, graft bridging, tendon advancement, balloon arthroplasty, superior capsular reconstruction, reverse total shoulder arthroplasty, among others [3]. Each of these treatment options have associated limitations and complications without one being clinically superior [3]. According to the American Academy of Orthopaedic Surgeons 2019 Management of Rotator Cuff Injuries Clinical Practice Guidelines, the authors did not find sufficient evidence to support the efficacy of any of the above surgical options; however, they do agree that they may improve patient reported outcomes [4].

A. Wilhelm · S. Akhavan (✉)
Orthopaedic Sports Medicine, Allegheny Health Network, Pittsburgh, PA, USA

C. Lavender (ed.), *Biologic and Nanoarthroscopic Approaches in Sports Medicine*, https://doi.org/10.1007/978-3-030-71323-2_9

Partial repair of the rotator cuff has been advocated whenever a complete repair cannot be completed to assist with balancing the coupled forces of the rotator cuff. Lee et al. recently showed that a partial repair of the rotator cuff improved clinical outcomes regardless of whether healing occured [5]. A 2020 systematic review showed that performing a partial repair in the setting of an irreparable massive rotator cuff tear resulted in a retear rate of 45% [3]. Revision surgery following partial repair was performed in about 10% of these patients. Mihata et al. showed that in patients who underwent both an SCR and partial cuff repair, the SCR prevented retear of the torn cuff at 1 year postoperatively and improved the quality of the repaired tendon on follow-up MRI [6].

The utilization of graft bridging or interposition in the setting of massive rotator cuff tears has been reported. This technique is performed by attaching the graft to the remaining cuff to "bridge" the gap in an irreducible rotator cuff repair. Graft interposition has demonstrated improvements in re-tear rates (20%) compared to partial tendon repair (45%) in massive irreparable cuff tears. Unfortunately, Graft interposition also resulted in twice as many revision operations [3, 7]. In a systematic review comparing graft bridging and SCR for large to massive cuff tears, Lin et al. found that both had improvements in clinical outcomes, with similar healing and complication rates [8]. In Mihata's original biomechanical study comparing bridge grafting versus SCR, he found that grafting to the torn tendon decreased superior humeral translation; however, it did not restore it back similar to that of an intact rotator cuff [1]. In the scenario of the SCR with fascia lata, there was complete restoration similar to an intact cuff. This led the authors to theorize that graft bridging may lead to a higher rate of re-tears due to increased subacromial impingement from lack of superior humeral stability.

Other options including muscle transfers, such as latissimus dorsi, lower trapezius, and other muscles, have been utilized for patients with an irreparable rotator cuff repair. The most commonly utilized techniques include an open two-incision and an arthroscopic-assisted transfer [3]. In massive irreparable tears, tendon transfers demonstrated a tendon transfer failure rate of about 15% [3]. A systematic review of the arthroscopic-assisted transfer procedure showed an overall complication rate of about 20% where complications included transfer failure, fracture, hematoma, deltoid deficiency, nerve dysesthesias, stiffness, among others [9]. The rate and severity of complications associated with tendon transfers are of concern compared to SCR.

Finally, reverse total shoulder arthroplasty (rTSA) has become an excellent option for an elderly patient with an irreparable rotator cuff tear, adequately relieving pain and restoring function of the shoulder [10]. In a systematic review by Petrillo et al., they address the intraoperative and perioperative complications which occur at a high rate, resulting in high revision rates [10]. In another systematic review of rTSA for massive irreparable cuff tears, they found a prosthesis failure rate of up to 10% [3]. The authors of this review believe that the use of rTSA should be employed in healthy, elderly patients with pseudoparalysis due to chronic irreparable massive tears. In the setting of a younger, more active patient, the utilization of joint preservation procedures should be sought.

The SCR was introduced to assist in this difficult problem and has the added benefit of being a joint preserving procedure. Since the introduction of the SCR, there have been a number of different technique variations and graft choices utilized [4]. The idea behind superior capsular reconstruction was first published by Dr. Mihata in 2012 after he proposed a technique to restore the superior capsule of the glenohumeral joint [1]. Patients with a massive irreparable rotator cuff tear will have a defect of the superior capsule which lies on the undersurface of the supraspinatus and infraspinatus tendons [11]. This superior capsule has been found to play a role in the superior stability of the glenohumeral joint in Dr. Mihata's original biomechanical cadaveric study [1]. Without the restraint of the rotator cuff and superior capsule, superior translation of the humerus occurs with resulting altered kinematics eventually leading to subacromial impingement and osseous changes [12]. A cadaveric study demonstrated that a defect in the superior capsule leads to an increase in glenohumeral translation in all directions [13]. Reconstruction of the superior capsule results in reversal of proximal humeral migration and optimization of the force couples about the shoulder complex [1, 11, 14].

2 Indications/Contraindications

The indications for a superior capsular reconstruction include a massive irreparable tear of the supraspinatus and/or infraspinatus, minimal to no glenohumeral arthritis, a functioning deltoid muscle, and an intact or reparable subscapularis tendon. If there is superior migration of the humerus preoperatively, there must be active reduction with inferior traction. The procedure can also be considered in patients with a failed rotator cuff repair who have significant underlying fatty infiltration evident on MRI, and intra-operatively there is concern for the tissue quality.

Contraindications to the superior capsular reconstruction include moderate to severe arthropathy of the glenohumeral joint (Hamada grade ≥ 3), torn or irreparable subscapularis, significant bony defects, significant shoulder stiffness, and absence of deltoid, latissimus dorsi, or pectoralis major function. Patients who are not medically fit to undergo surgery or those who will not follow the postoperative rehabilitation protocol should not undergo this procedure as well.

3 Surgical Technique

3.1 Positioning and Diagnostic Arthroscopy

This technique can be performed in the lateral decubitus or the beach chair position; however, the authors preferred the beach chair position. The arm is held in an arm holder which allows for inferior traction to assist with creating a subacromial space along with rotation to allow easier placement of anchors. Standard anterior, posterior, and lateral arthroscopy portals are used; however, our posterior portal is placed slightly superior to allow visualization above the humerus. The lateral portal is made larger to allow passage of graft and freedom to reach both anterior and posterior. Neviaser portal is utilized to allow placement of the central glenoid anchor. Accessory portals are used for humeral anchor placement and occasionally for the anterior and posterior glenoid anchors.

The posterior viewing portal is utilized with a 30-degree arthroscope and a thorough diagnostic intra-articular evaluation is performed. At this point, attention is focused on the integrity of the subscapularis and biceps. If there is a tear or partial tear of the subscapularis identified, this is addressed at that time. If biceps pathology is identified, it is addressed with either a biceps tenotomy or tenodesis as indicated/preferred.

Tips and Pearls – Portal Placement (1) Place the superior portal higher than for a standard intra-articular arthroscopy to allow unimpeded viewing of the entire subacromial space. If the portal is too low and anterior viewing is difficult due to the humeral head, a supero-lateral viewing portal can be used. (2) Center the lateral portal on the rotator cuff tear to allow easy access to the front and back of the humeral head. This will be important to allow repair of the posterior rotator cuff to the graft. (3) The anterior portal can be used for anterior anchor placement on the glenoid. In order to do so, it must be laterally and superiorly placed to allow for an appropriate angle for placement.

3.2 Subacromial Debridement

We will then move to the subacromial space where a bursectomy will be performed allowing for better visualization of the rotator cuff. If needed, an acromioplasty will be performed at this time as well. Careful evaluation of the supraspinatus and infraspinatus is performed, paying attention to tissue quality, tear size, retraction distance, mobility, and sites of adhesions. All efforts will be made to perform direct repair of the rotator cuff including interval slides as indicated. At this point, after full mobilization of the rotator cuff, if the cuff cannot be fully repaired, we will proceed with SCR using acellular dermal allograft (Fig. 1) (Arthrex Inc. Naples, Fl). In preparation of the SCR, a debridement is performed in order to adequately visualize the medial glenoid, the posterior cuff, and laterally over the humerus for placement of lateral row fixation.

3.3 Anchor Placement

In order to provide an adequate bony surface on the glenoid for the graft, the superior labrum is fully removed, ensuring to have bony exposure at least 5–10 mm medially from the edge of the glenoid. This will also be helpful to allow visualization during anchor placement. Three glenoid anchors are placed (3.9 mm Knotless Corkscrew; Arthrex Inc., Naples, FL). The anterior anchor is placed at the base of the coracoid, generally through the anterior portal. An accessory portal just anterior

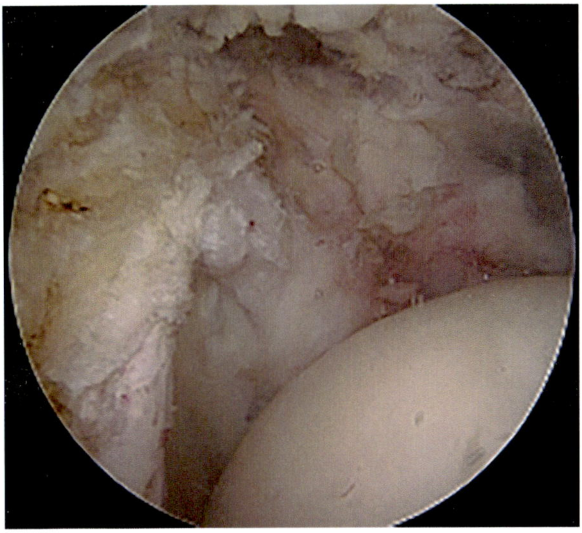

Fig. 1 Right shoulder, posterior viewing portal. Massive rotator cuff tear with retraction medial to the glenoid face. No significant glenohumeral arthrosis is noted. The long head of the biceps has already been addressed

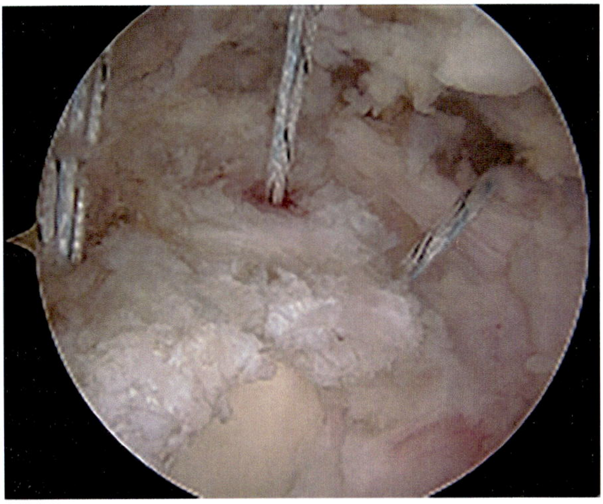

Fig. 2 Right shoulder, posterior viewing portal. The middle glenoid anchor was placed through a Neviaser portal

to the acromion can be used if the trajectory through the anterior portal is inadequate. The posterior anchor is placed through the posterior portal while viewing from the lateral position. Again, an accessory portal may be utilized. Finally, a central anchor is placed through the Neviaser portal, positioned between the anterior and posterior anchors. It is imperative to ensure that you are medial enough to avoid the penetration of the articular surface, yet lateral enough to not endanger the suprascapular nerve as seen in Fig. 2.

Pearls (1) Keep sutures from glenoid anchors in respective portals to assist with suture management. (2) Ensure that middle anchor placement is medial enough to

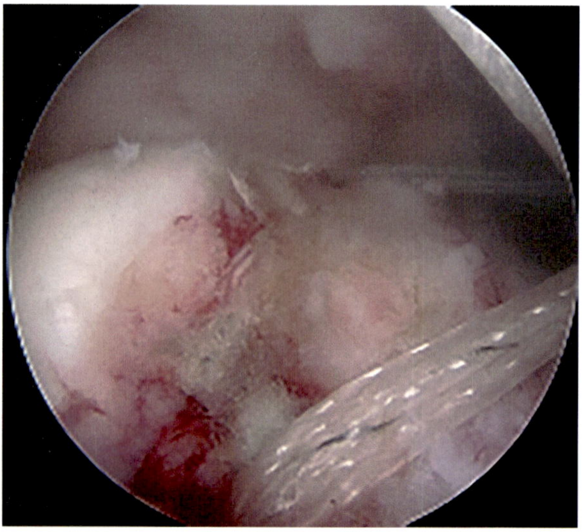

Fig. 3 Right shoulder, posterior viewing portal. Placement of the two medial row anchors in the humerus, just lateral to the articular margin

avoid penetration of articular surface, yet lateral enough from scapular spine to avoid suprascapular nerve.

The next step begins with preparing the bone bed of the greater tuberosity of the humerus, which is completed with use of motorized shaver, electrocautery, and/or burr. Two or three (depending on the size of the tear) medial anchors are placed in the humerus at the junction of the articular cartilage through accessory percutaneous holes. The anchors are cannulated threaded anchors (4.75 mm BioComposite SwiveLock; Arthrex) which are preloaded with a braded suture tape (FiberTape; Arthrex). The anterior anchor is placed just posterior to the biceps groove, while the posterior anchor is placed at the posterior aspect of the cuff tear as seen in Fig. 3. An additional anchor can be placed in between these two anchors if the cuff tear is large. Maintain the sutures in these accessory holes to assist with suture management. Once the medial anchors of the humerus are placed, we then insert a PassPort Button cannula (Arthrex) into the lateral portal.

Pearls (1) Maintain the medial row anchor sutures within the percutaneous accessory holes to assist with suture management. (2) Insert PassPort Button cannula into lateral portal after the medial row anchors have been inserted.

3.4 Graft Preparation

The typical graft used for this procedure is an acellular dermal allograft which is 3.0 mm thick (ArthroFLEX; Arthrex). A calibrated probe is used to measure the distance between the anchors (Fig. 4). We start with grabbing the sutures from the

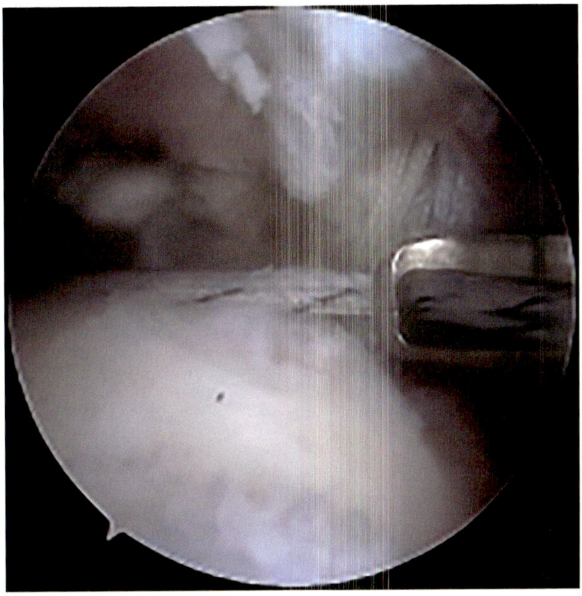

Fig. 4 Right shoulder, posterior viewing portal. Use of the calibrated probe to determine the distance between anchors

anterior humeral anchor, and while using the calibrated probe, we measure to the anterior glenoid anchor and then to the posterior humeral anchor. We then take the suture from the posterior glenoid and measure to the anterior glenoid anchor, ensuring we are following the contour of the glenoid, and to the posterior humeral anchor. Using these measurements, we draw out our needed graft size on the back table and mark the locations of the anchors on the graft. We add 10 mm to each end of the graft in the medial to lateral direction to help prevent suture cutout and add 15 mm in the anterior/posterior direction to ensure coverage of the footprint. Sharp scissors are used to cut our graft to size.

Tips and Pearls Standard measurements are to add 10 mm between each anchor anterior to posterior and 15 mm from medial to lateral. If increased tension in the graft is desired, 5 mm can be added between each anchor and 10 mm medial to lateral. To pass the humeral anchor fibertapes through the graft, a punch is used to create holes to assist with channeling of the suture during passage of the graft. The graft is then brought up to the patient's arm and may either be held by an assistant or placed on a towel on the arm. The two FiberTape sutures are brought out of the PassPort Button cannula and placed through the punched holes in their respective position. It is imperative to maintain orientation of the graft during these steps.

Tips and Pearls In order to keep the fibertapes inferior in the cannula, an Opsite can be used and the fibertapes can be stuck to the arm inferiorly.

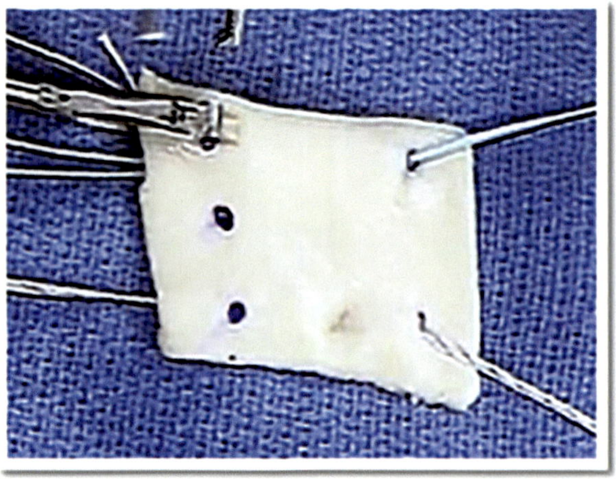

Fig. 5 ArthroFLEX graft with anchor locations marked, passing glenoid repair stitch using Scorpion

3.5 Suture Retrieval and Passage

From one glenoid anchor at a time, we retrieve the repair stitch and the loop side of the shuttle stitch out of the PassPort cannula. Utilizing an antegrade suture passer (FastPass Scorpion; Arthrex), pass the repair stitch in a mattress configuration over its corresponding anchor position as seen in Fig. 5. The repair stitch is then passed through the loop of the shuttle stitch and the free end of the shuttle stitch is pulled, passing the repair stitch through the anchor and out of the original portal. This step is repeated for all three glenoid anchors, ensuring no suture entanglement during passing.

3.6 Graft Passage

At this point, we are ready to pass the graft into the shoulder through the PassPort Button cannula. Use an Alice Clamp or grasper at the leading edge of the graft and insert the graft into the cannula. Sequentially apply tension on the three repair stitches from the glenoid anchors while inserting the graft into the shoulder. Any slack from the FiberTape should be removed during insertion as well. Continue to pull the glenoid repair stitches until the graft has been tensioned appropriately to the glenoid neck bone bed as seen in Fig. 6. Once this has been achieved, we look under the graft to ensure there is no slack remaining as we apply tension to the lateral sutures. The repair stitches can be cut with an arthroscopic cutter. If we believe there are any dog ears that will form to the graft with final fixation, we will use the Scorpion to pass individual suture tapes (SutureTape Link; Arthrex) where appropriate to tie into our lateral row (Fig. 7). A SpeedBridge technique is completed at this time using two lateral anchors (4.75 mm SwiveLock; Arthrex), crisscrossing the FiberTapes. Re-evaluation of the tension and fixation can be completed at this time, with extra anchors placed into the humerus or glenoid as needed.

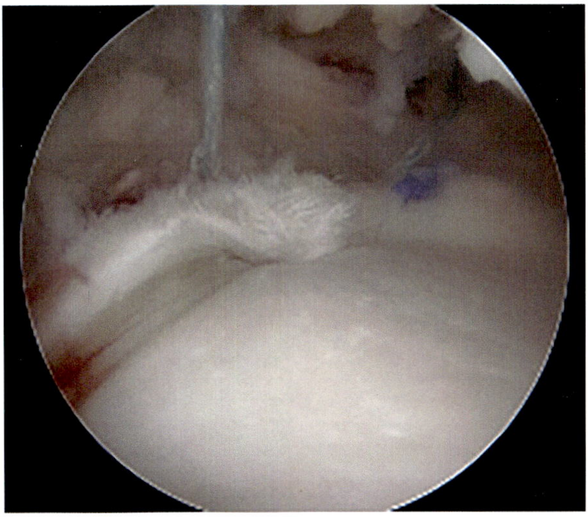

Fig. 6 Right shoulder, posterior viewing portal. Dermal allograft reduced into position on glenoid neck

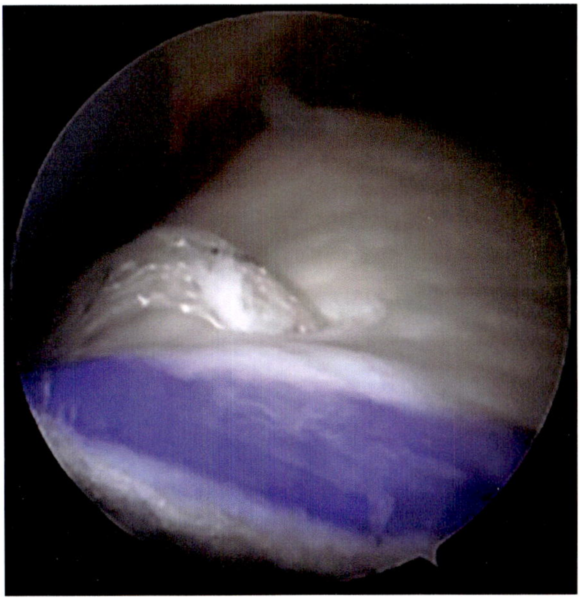

Fig. 7 Left shoulder, posterior viewing portal. FiberTapes of humeral medial row passing through reduced graft, prior to SpeedBridge fixation

Pearls (1) Do not twist graft when inserting into cannula. (2) Remove slack from all sutures as passing graft. (3) May add suture tape to help prevent dog ears to graft.

As a final step, the remaining posterior rotator cuff is repaired to the posterior dermal graft as seen in Fig. 8. This can be accomplished with the use of the Scorpion or SutureLasso. It is our experience that it is critical to change the Scorpion needle prior to passing sutures in this step, as the original needle has been dulled with its

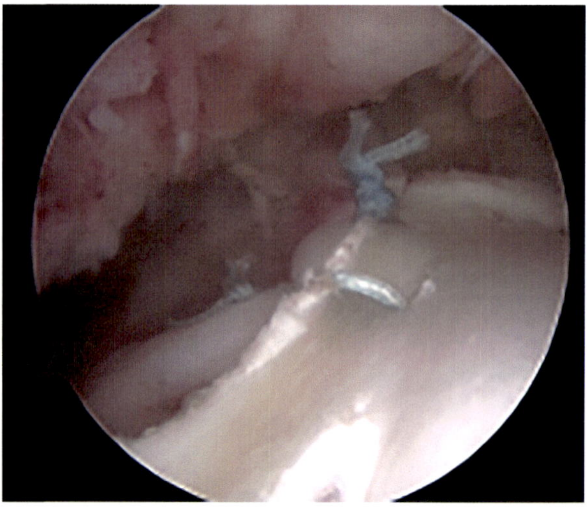

Fig. 8 Right shoulder, lateral viewing portal. Posterior cuff has been repaired to the posterior graft

multiple prior passes through the graft. We pass all required sutures first and then tie an arthroscopic sliding knot. If there is remaining rotator interval tissue anteriorly, the graft can be repaired to this as well. It is important to not repair the anterior graft to the subscapularis, as this will restrict motion. Final images are taken as the procedure is now complete. The patient is placed into a bump sling post-op. Postoperative rehabilitation protocol of this patient is the same as for a large rotator cuff repair. Patients are limited to a passive range of motion for the first 6 weeks, active motion is initiated thereafter, and finally at the 12-week mark strengthening exercises are initiated.

Pearls (1) Exchange the Scorpion needle if using this to pass sutures in this step. (2) Do not repair the anterior graft to the subscapularis tendon.

3.7 Partial Rotator Cuff Repair Over the SCR

It is our experience that once the graft has been reduced to the glenoid and tension has been applied to the lateral sutures, depression of the humeral head will have occurred. Due to this, we find that the residual cuff tissue may have improved excursion toward the greater tuberosity footprint due to improved acromiohumeral distance. If there is enough excursion of the cuff at this point, we will perform a partial repair on top of the graft. The FiberTape sutures which have passed through the graft will be separated into four individual strands and then passed through the retracted cuff tissue using a Scorpion. We will then perform the SpeedBridge technique using two lateral anchors as described previously. Figures 9 and 10 show the final product of this technique with the cuff reduced

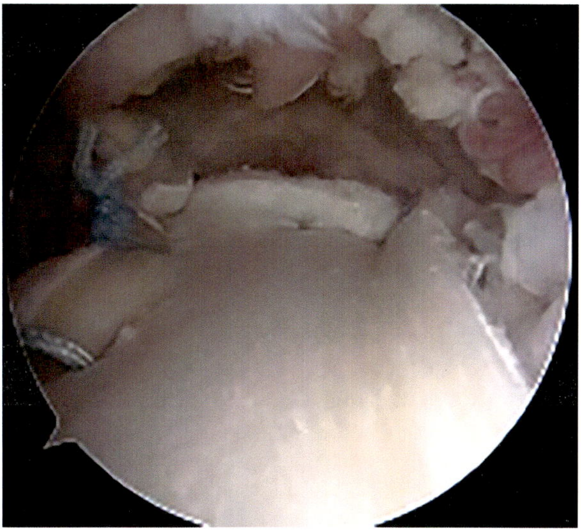

Fig. 9 Right shoulder, lateral viewing portal. SCR is completed

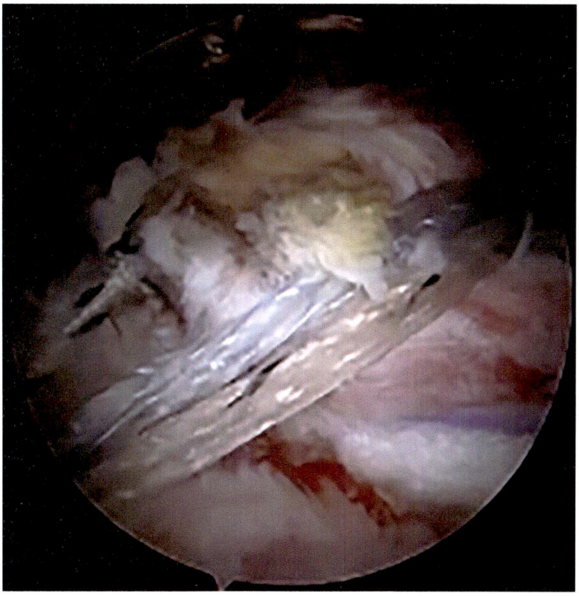

Fig. 10 Left shoulder, lateral viewing portal. Dermal allograft is seen covered by a partial repair of the rotator cuff over the top. Also demonstrated is the use of a FiberLink assisting in reducing the dermal graft to the humeral footprint

over the top of the dermal graft. We do not alter our postoperative protocol if this extra step is performed.

4 Discussion

During the years 2007–2009 when Dr. Mihata initially performed the superior capsular reconstruction procedure on his patients, he had excellent patient-related outcomes. In the 24 shoulders that he performed this procedure on, there was an increase in mean active elevation from 84 degrees to 148 degrees, almost a doubling of the acromiohumeral distance, and a significant improvement in the American Shoulder and Elbow Surgeons (ASES) score at around 3 years post-operatively [11]. In his surgical technique, he reconstructed the superior capsule, attaching a fascia lata autograft from the superior glenoid to the greater tuberosity of the humerus. He found superior results biomechanically when attaching the graft to the glenoid versus the remaining rotator cuff tissue [1, 11].

Shortly after the publication of his case series, other surgeons began to utilize his surgical technique and even altered it slightly. In 2015, Hirahara and Adams were the first to publish a SCR technique utilizing a dermal allograft followed by doctors Burkhart and Petri separately the following year [15–17]. Others have suggested the utilization of the long head of the biceps tendon as an available, local tissue autograft [18, 19]. Subsequent studies and systematic reviews have shown good to excellent short-term clinical outcomes with adequate pain relief and functional improvement [16, 20].

The use of allograft has gained popularity as it has the advantage of no donor site morbidity, shorter surgical times, ease of preparation, and potential strength of the graft [15]. There are multiple different allograft options available to surgeons at this time, including acellular human dermal tissue, porcine small intestine submucosa, bovine dermis, equine pericardium, Teflon felt, among others [15, 21, 22]. Given the increased use of human dermal allograft with successful short-term results in the United States, Mihata et al. compared the biomechanical differences between this graft and a fascia lata allograft [23]. Both graft options restored superior glenohumeral joint forces and subacromial contact characteristics, likely resulting in relief of clinical subacromial impingement symptoms. The human dermal allograft however only restored about 50% of the superior glenohumeral stability with increased humeral head translation, whereas the fascia lata restored this completely. The study also demonstrated lengthening of the dermal allograft by about 15% whereas the fascia lata graft did not show any lengthening. These differences may be due to many factors including the thickness of the graft.

In the biomechanical study comparing dermal allograft versus fascia lata allograft, Mihata et al. found that suturing of the posterior cuff to the posterior graft should be performed at minimum in both reconstruction techniques [23]. With human dermal allograft, they found that isolated posterior anchoring resulted in significantly increased glenohumeral motion relative to an intact rotator cuff. Adding anterior anchoring with fascia lata grafting only resulted in restricted overall shoulder motion. This led to their recommendation of only posterior attachment with fascia lata grafting, while human dermal allograft should be anchored both anterior and posterior. Hirahara et al. have demonstrated improved ASES scores postoperatively when the human dermal allograft is anchored both anteriorly and posteriorly [24].

A systematic review comparing autograft versus allograft in SCR found that both graft options improved clinical outcomes, with the graft tear rates appearing similar [25]. A systematic review by Altintas et al. have found similar positive results regardless of graft type chosen [20]. There are multiple systematic reviews which have demonstrated higher rates of re-tear within the human dermal allografts versus fascia lata grafts; however, they are not statistically significant [3, 26, 27]. The thickness of the dermal graft can also determine outcomes. Mihata et al. demonstrated superior biomechanical outcomes with an eight-millimeter graft when compared to a 4-mm graft [14, 28]. Hirahara et al. found that grafts greater than 3 mm had significantly better results compared to smaller grafts [24]. Of interesting note, the maximal thickness of available allografts is only 3–4 mm [20].

The lack of thicker available autografts has led some authors to consider variations in the surgical technique of the SCR. Curtis et al. performed a biomechanical study to evaluate the use of a dermal autograft on the undersurface of the acromion in addition to the standard SCR with dermal autograft. They found that the additional graft resulted in decreased superior humeral head translation compared to the standard SCR; however, we did note non-significant increases in subacromial contact pressures relative to an intact rotator cuff [29]. It is undetermined what effects the increased subacromial contact pressures would have clinically.

The term pseudoparalysis has been used to describe patients whose pain-free maximum active forward elevation is less than or equal to 90 degrees with preserved passive motion in the setting of a rotator cuff tear [30]. Reversal of true pseudoparalysis was thought to only be accomplished by a reverse total shoulder arthroplasty; however, Burkhart and Mihata have both demonstrated that this can be accomplished with the SCR as well [30, 31]. Burkhart believes that with evidence of comparable short-term results to rTSA, and if the SCR is not durable long term, the rTSA remains a viable option [30]. To date, the longest follow-up data for the SCR procedure is a 5-year follow-up study of 30 patients by Mihata et al. [32]. Their findings show significant improvement in ASES, active elevation, and acromiohumeral distance at both 1 and 5 years compared to pre-operatively. The ASES scores were significantly higher at 5 years compared to 1-year post-op. At 5-year post-op, 92% of patients returned to previous physical work and 100% returned to prior sports. Of importance, only patients who had torn grafts (3) progressed onto cuff arthropathy in this mid-term follow-up study. It is still to be determined how the SCR will perform long term. Sochacki et al. summarized in their systematic review that, "Arthroscopic SCR for massive irreparable rotator cuff tears results in statistically significant and clinically significant improvement in patient-reported outcomes and shoulder ROM with low graft failure, complication, and reoperation rate." [33].

Complications related to the superior capsular reconstruction in its short-term follow-up have been limited. The rate of graft tearing, which is the most common complication from this procedure, occurred at a pooled rate around 3.8–13%; however, it has been reported to be as high as 75% [3, 20, 33]. Following an SCR, the overall revision surgery rate is around 5% [3]. The most common location of graft tearing was from the humerus [20]. Other less common complications reported following an SCR include shoulder stiffness, infection, and anchor/suture pullout. Although the complication and revision rates for rTSA in massive cuff tears appear to be decreasing (12% major complication, 5% minor complication, 1.4% revision), the major complications (acromial fracture, dislocation, baseplate failures) involved outweigh those involved with SCR [20, 34].

In summary, the superior capsular reconstruction appears to be a viable option for a difficult clinical situation. This joint-preserving procedure has shown promising short-term patient-related outcomes with minimal overall risks. Over the next decade, it is imperative to pay close attention to the long-term outcomes and the ideal patient population for this procedure.

5 Editor's View

This technique has dramatically changed my clinical practice for difficult-to-repair and irreparable rotator cuffs. The results of the procedure are very promising for a condition that was notorious for poor outcomes. Patients who are not ready or eligible for joint reconstructions now have a great option to restore function and pain in this setting. I always say not to do a joint reconstruction for a soft tissue issue. Try to preserve at all costs and this technique certainly helps us do that.

References

1. Mihata T, McGarry M, Pirolo J. Superior capsule reconstruction to restore superior stability in irreparable rotator cuff tears: a biomechanical cadaveric study. Am J Sports Med. 2012;40(10):2248–55. https://doi.org/10.1177/0363546512456195.
2. Bedi ADJ, Warren R, et al. Massive tears of the rotator cuff. J Bone Joint Surg Am. 2010;92(9):1894–908. https://doi.org/10.2106/JBJS.I.01531.
3. Kovacevic DSR, Grawe B, et al. Management of irreparable massive rotator cuff tears: a systematic review and meta-analysis of patient-reported outcomes, reoperation rates and treatment response. J Shoulder Elb Surg. 2020;4(S1058-2746(20)30624-8) https://doi.org/10.1016/j.jse.2020.07.030.
4. Weber S, Chahal J. Management of Rotator Cuff Injuries. J Am Acad Orthop Surg. 2020;28(5):e193–201. https://doi.org/10.5435/JAAOS-D-19-00463.
5. Lee KW, Lee GS, Yang DS, Park SH, Chun YS, Choy WS. Clinical outcome of arthroscopic partial repair of large to massive posterosuperior rotator cuff tears: medialization of the attachment site of the rotator cuff tendon. Clin Orthop Surg. 2020;12(3):353–63. https://doi.org/10.4055/cios19126.
6. Mihata T, Lee TQ, Hasegawa A, Fukunishi K, Kawakami T, Fujisawa Y, et al. Superior capsule reconstruction for reinforcement of arthroscopic rotator cuff repair improves cuff integrity. Am J Sports Med. 2019;47(2):379–88. https://doi.org/10.1177/0363546518816689.
7. Mori D, Funakoshi N, Yamashita F. Arthroscopic surgery of irreparable large or massive rotator cuff tears with low-grade fatty degeneration of the infraspinatus: patch autograft procedure versus partial repair procedure. Arthroscopy. 2013;29(12):1911–21. https://doi.org/10.1016/j.arthro.2013.08.032.

8. Lin J, Sun Y, Chen Q, Liu S, Ding Z, Chen J. Outcome comparison of graft bridging and superior capsule reconstruction for large to massive rotator cuff tears: a systematic review. Am J Sports Med. 2020;48(11):2828–38. https://doi.org/10.1177/0363546519889040.
9. Osti L, Buda M, Andreotti M, Gerace E, Osti R, Massari L, et al. Arthroscopic-assisted latissimus dorsi transfer for massive rotator cuff tear: a systematic review. Br Med Bull. 2018;128(1):23–35. https://doi.org/10.1093/bmb/ldy030.
10. Petrillo S, Longo UG, Papalia R, Denaro V. Reverse shoulder arthroplasty for massive irreparable rotator cuff tears and cuff tear arthropathy: a systematic review. Musculoskelet Surg. 2017;101(2):105–12. https://doi.org/10.1007/s12306-017-0474-z.
11. Mihata T, Lee TQ, Watanabe C, Fukunishi K, Ohue M, Tsujimura T, et al. Clinical results of arthroscopic superior capsule reconstruction for irreparable rotator cuff tears. Arthroscopy. 2013;29(3):459–70. https://doi.org/10.1016/j.arthro.2012.10.022.
12. Duralde XA, Bair B. Massive rotator cuff tears: the result of partial rotator cuff repair. J Shoulder Elb Surg. 2005;14(2):121–7. https://doi.org/10.1016/j.jse.2004.06.015.
13. Ishihara Y, Mihata T, Tamboli M, Nguyen L, Park KJ, McGarry MH, et al. Role of the superior shoulder capsule in passive stability of the glenohumeral joint. J Shoulder Elb Surg. 2014;23(5):642–8. https://doi.org/10.1016/j.jse.2013.09.025.
14. Mihata T, McGarry MH, Kahn T, Goldberg I, Neo M, Lee TQ. Biomechanical effect of thickness and tension of fascia lata graft on glenohumeral stability for superior capsule reconstruction in irreparable supraspinatus tears. Arthroscopy. 2016;32(3):418–26. https://doi.org/10.1016/j.arthro.2015.08.024.
15. Hirahara AM, Adams CR. Arthroscopic superior capsular reconstruction for treatment of massive irreparable rotator cuff tears. Arthrosc Tech. 2015;4(6):e637–41. https://doi.org/10.1016/j.eats.2015.07.006.
16. Burkhart SS, Denard PJ, Adams CR, Brady PC, Hartzler RU. Arthroscopic superior capsular reconstruction for massive irreparable rotator cuff repair. Arthrosc Tech. 2016;5(6):e1407–e18. https://doi.org/10.1016/j.eats.2016.08.024.
17. Petri M, Greenspoon JA, Millett PJ. Arthroscopic superior capsule reconstruction for irreparable rotator cuff tears. Arthrosc Tech. 2015;4(6):e751–5. https://doi.org/10.1016/j.eats.2015.07.018.
18. Boutsiadis A, Chen S, Jiang C, Lenoir H, Delsol P, Barth J. Long head of the biceps as a suitable available local tissue autograft for superior capsular reconstruction: "The Chinese Way". Arthrosc Tech. 2017;6(5):e1559–e66. https://doi.org/10.1016/j.eats.2017.06.030.
19. El-Shaar R, Soin S, Nicandri G, Maloney M, Voloshin I. Superior capsular reconstruction with a long head of the biceps tendon autograft: a cadaveric study. Orthop J Sports Med. 2018;6(7):2325967118785365. https://doi.org/10.1177/2325967118785365.
20. Altintas B, Scheidt M, Kremser V, Boykin R, Bhatia S, Sajadi KR, et al. Superior capsule reconstruction for irreparable massive rotator cuff tears: does it make sense? A systematic review of early clinical evidence. Am J Sports Med. 2020;363546520904378 https://doi.org/10.1177/0363546520904378.
21. Gabler C, Spohn J, Tischer T, Bader R. Biomechanical, biochemical, and cell biological evaluation of different collagen scaffolds for tendon augmentation. Biomed Res Int. 2018;2018:7246716. https://doi.org/10.1155/2018/7246716.
22. Okamura K, Abe M, Yamada Y, Makihara T, Yoshimizu T, Sakaki Y, et al. Arthroscopic superior capsule reconstruction with Teflon felt synthetic graft for irreparable massive rotator cuff tears: clinical and radiographic results at minimum 2-year follow-up. J Shoulder Elb Surg. 2020; https://doi.org/10.1016/j.jse.2020.06.022.
23. Mihata T, Bui CNH, Akeda M, Cavagnaro MA, Kuenzler M, Peterson AB, et al. A biomechanical cadaveric study comparing superior capsule reconstruction using fascia lata allograft with human dermal allograft for irreparable rotator cuff tear. J Shoulder Elb Surg. 2017;26(12):2158–66. https://doi.org/10.1016/j.jse.2017.07.019.
24. Hirahara AM, Andersen WJ, Panero AJ. Superior capsular reconstruction: clinical outcomes after minimum 2-year follow-up. Am J Orthop (Belle Mead NJ). 2017;46(6):266–78.

25. Kim DM, Shin MJ, Kim H, Park D, Jeon IH, Kholinne E, et al. Comparison between autografts and allografts in superior capsular reconstruction: a systematic review of outcomes. Orthop J Sports Med. 2020;8(3):2325967120904937. https://doi.org/10.1177/2325967120904937.
26. de Campos Azevedo CI, Andrade R, Leiria Pires Gago Angelo AC, Espregueira-Mendes J, Ferreira N, Sevivas N. Fascia lata autograft versus human dermal allograft in arthroscopic superior capsular reconstruction for irreparable rotator cuff tears: a systematic review of clinical outcomes. Arthroscopy. 2020;36(2):579–91 e2. https://doi.org/10.1016/j.arthro.2019.08.033.
27. Abd Elrahman AA, Sobhy MH, Abdelazim H, Omar Haroun HK. Superior capsular reconstruction: fascia lata versus acellular dermal allograft: a systematic review. Arthrosc Sports Med Rehabil. 2020;2(4):e389–e97. https://doi.org/10.1016/j.asmr.2020.03.002.
28. Denard PJ, Brady PC, Adams CR, Tokish JM, Burkhart SS. Preliminary results of arthroscopic superior capsule reconstruction with dermal allograft. Arthroscopy. 2018;34(1):93–9. https://doi.org/10.1016/j.arthro.2017.08.265.
29. Curtis DM, Lee CS, Qin C, Edgington J, Parekh A, Miller J, et al. Superior capsule reconstruction with subacromial allograft spacer: biomechanical cadaveric study of subacromial contact pressure and superior humeral head translation. Arthroscopy. 2020;36(3):680–6. https://doi.org/10.1016/j.arthro.2019.09.047.
30. Burkhart SS, Hartzler RU. Superior capsular reconstruction reverses profound pseudoparalysis in patients with irreparable rotator cuff tears and minimal or no glenohumeral arthritis. Arthroscopy. 2019;35(1):22–8. https://doi.org/10.1016/j.arthro.2018.07.023.
31. Mihata T, Lee TQ, Hasegawa A, Kawakami T, Fukunishi K, Fujisawa Y, et al. Arthroscopic superior capsule reconstruction can eliminate pseudoparalysis in patients with irreparable rotator cuff tears. Am J Sports Med. 2018;46(11):2707–16. https://doi.org/10.1177/0363546518786489.
32. Mihata T, Lee TQ, Hasegawa A, Fukunishi K, Kawakami T, Fujisawa Y, et al. Five-year follow-up of arthroscopic superior capsule reconstruction for irreparable rotator cuff tears. J Bone Joint Surg Am. 2019;101(21):1921–30. https://doi.org/10.2106/JBJS.19.00135.
33. Sochacki KR, McCulloch PC, Lintner DM, Harris JD. Superior capsular reconstruction for massive rotator cuff tear leads to significant improvement in range of motion and clinical outcomes: a systematic review. Arthroscopy. 2019;35(4):1269–77. https://doi.org/10.1016/j.arthro.2018.10.129.
34. Hartzler RU, Steen BM, Hussey MM, Cusick MC, Cottrell BJ, Clark RE, et al. Reverse shoulder arthroplasty for massive rotator cuff tear: risk factors for poor functional improvement. J Shoulder Elb Surg. 2015;24(11):1698–706. https://doi.org/10.1016/j.jse.2015.04.015.

Treatment of Osteochondritis Dissecans of the Elbow with BioCartilage

Sohaib Malik and Charles Giangarra

1 Introduction

Osteochondritis dissecans (OCD) of the elbow is a condition seen in adolescent overhead athletes causing chondral and subchondral damage to the capitellum. Repetitive overhead actions corresponding to throwing, gymnastics, and weightlifting trigger microtrauma because of axial loading and shear on the radiocapitellar articulation which could cause fragmentation, resorption, and lack of subchondral bone and, in later stages, cartilage fractures with loose bodies within the joint [1]. The reported incidence of OCD in adolescent baseball players is 1.3–3.4% [2]. The affected person normally presents with insidious onset of elbow pain that is worse with exercise and may additionally have a flexion contracture, posterolateral swelling, and lateral elbow pain upon valgus stress. Radiographs of the elbow may illustrate subchondral lucency, and in later stages, loose bodies within the joint. MRI is beneficial for evaluating the size of the lesion in addition to the integrity of the cartilage cap. Treatment of the lesion is guided by an assessment of the lesion's stability, which is predicated on the integrity of the cartilage cap, presence or absence of mechanical symptoms, and loss of range of motion.

A variety of treatment strategies addressing OCD lesions of the capitellum have been described, including open reduction internal fixation, fragment excision with microfracture, and osteochondral transplantation [2]. Size and stability of the lesion dictate the optimal treatment regimen, although risks and benefits of various techniques do not yield a single optimal plan for each case, as it must be tailored to the patient. These procedures can be performed through open lateral approaches or

S. Malik (✉)
Orthopedic Surgery Resident, Marshall University, Huntington, WV, USA

C. Giangarra
Department of Orthopaedic Surgery, VA Medical Center, Marshall University School of Medicine, Huntington, WV, USA

C. Lavender (ed.), *Biologic and Nanoarthroscopic Approaches in Sports Medicine*, https://doi.org/10.1007/978-3-030-71323-2_10

arthroscopically. A recent development in the treatment of OCD lesions in the knee and talus has been to use BioCartilage (Arthrex, Naples, FL), an FDA-regulated, dehydrated cartilage allograft that is placed over the lesion and sealed to augment cartilage healing after microfracture [3]. This dehydrated, human articular cartilage allograft serves as a scaffold to augment microfracture and has been shown in animal models to have increased proteoglycan and type II collagen, similar to hyaline articular cartilage, when compared to microfracture alone, which produces a fibrocartilage cap [4]. BioCartilage has shown promising clinical and MRI outcomes at short-term for talar OCD lesions compared to microfracture [5], and has recently shown to have good 2-year outcomes when used for chondral defects in the knee [6].

2 Indications/Contraindications

For an OCD lesion of the capitellum, indications for the BioCartilage implantation include an unstable type I lesion as well as a stable type II lesion. Indications for the use of BioCartilage are similar to that of microfracture: unstable lesions that, after debridement, have a stable rim. Contraindications for the use of BioCartilage include large fragments that can be fixed with bioabsorbable screws as well as early signs of osteoarthritis. Nonoperative treatment with rest and cessation of all overhead activities is the most common treatment for stable lesions (no mechanical symptoms, full ROM, stable cartilage cap), and disruption of the cartilage cap from the subchondral bone usually warrants surgical intervention.

3 Operative Technique

3.1 Positioning and Approach

We prefer to position the patient supine with the operative extremity on an arm board. A tourniquet is used. A standard lateral approach to the elbow is used to access the radiocapitellar joint. The joint is evaluated and any loose bodies are removed. The capitellar lesion is then visualized and debrided to a stable rim (Fig. 1).

3.2 Microfracture and BioCartilage

With the use of the microfracture awls, the subchondral bone at the base of the lesion was penetrated using microfracture technique. After microfracture a 1 mm vial of BioCartilage (Arthrex, Naples, FL) was prepared for usage. The BioCartilage was then mixed with 1 mm of the patient's own platelet-rich plasma and placed in the base of the lesion and was sealed with fibrin glue (Fig. 2). After filling and glue solidifying the elbow was taken through passive range of motion to confirm no interference with the elbow range of motion. The wound was then irrigated with

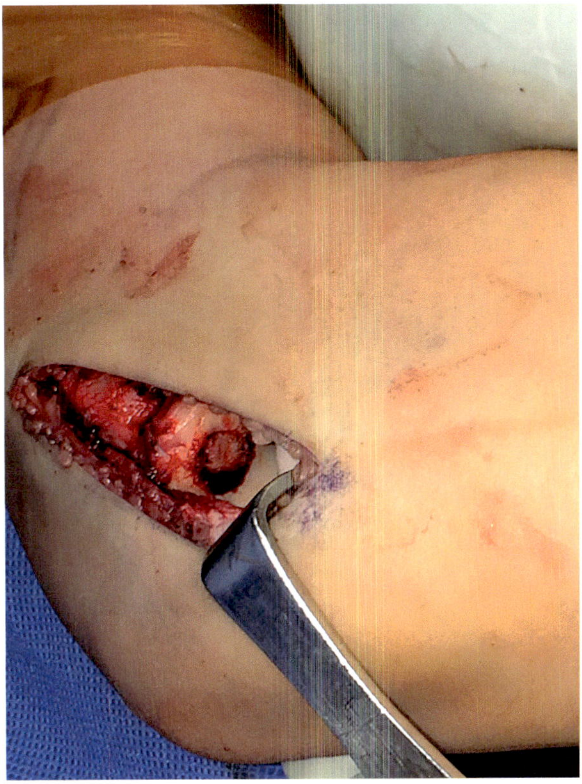

Fig. 1 Capitellum lesion visualized with circumferential edges and clear from any remaining cartilage

antibiotic-impregnated solution and closure of the capsule and superficial soft tissue was undertaken in the normal fashion and a sterile dressing was applied. The arm was then placed in a long-arm posterior splint at 90 degrees of flexion.

4 Discussion

Although microfracture alone has shown favorable short-term results, multiple studies with long-term follow up have shown patients with clinical and radiographic signs and symptoms of arthritis. Takahara et al. in 1999 reported that 46% of operatively treated OCD lesions had residual symptoms at a mean follow up of 12.6 years [7]. This is likely due to the formation of fibrocartilage, which is thought to be less durable than native hyaline cartilage. By restoring a more hyaline-like cartilage using BioCartilage allograft, more durable cartilage can cover the lesion without the donor-site morbidity of autologous osteochondral transfer.

Osteochondral autograft transfer has shown good results in elbow OCD lesions; however, there is some risk of donor-site morbidity, usually a nonarticular portion of the knee, which is avoided by using BioCartilage. Vogt et al. in 2011 reported on a series of 8 patients treated with OATs of the elbow, 6 of which had capitellum

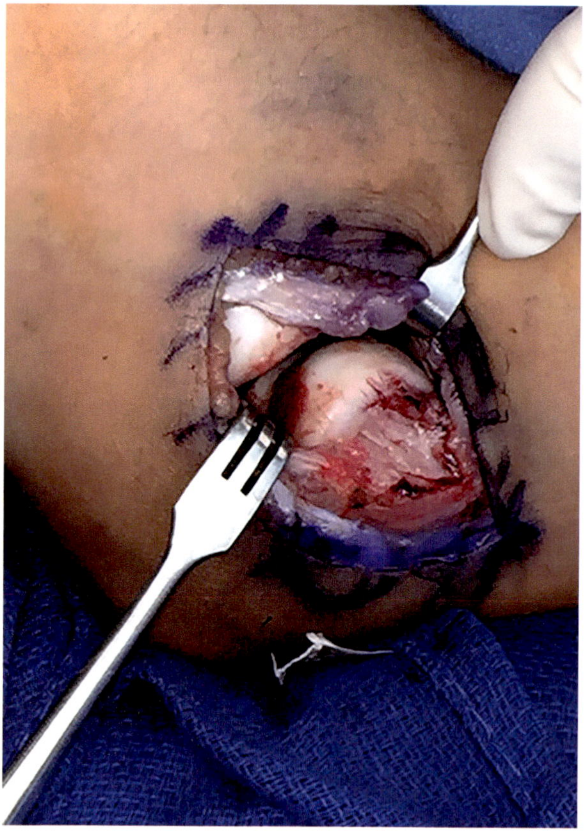

Fig. 2 Lesion has been prepared and you can see the BioCartilage has been glued into place

lesions, with an average of 10 years follow up [8]. They found that at a final follow up all patients had full extension and flexion matching the contralateral elbow with grade 1 K-L osteoarthritis in 2 patients. MRI showed integration of the graft in each patient. Subchondral cysts and edema found on MRI did not correlate with patients' clinical symptoms. Three patients complained of donor-site knee pain.

OCD lesions can be treated operatively by either open or arthroscopic means. Caldwell has described a technique for arthroscopic BioCartilage implantation. Although there is a trend toward minimally invasive surgery in all facets of orthopedics, we believe that an open approach to elbow OCD lesions is still a very useful operation. The technical challenges of elbow arthroscopy limit its ubiquity. At our academic institution elbow arthroscopy is an infrequent procedure. However, the lateral approach to the elbow joint should be able to be reliably performed by any competent orthopedic surgeon, which would benefit patients from potentially having to travel potentially long distances to be treated by a surgeon who specializes in elbow arthroscopy, saving time, money, and hassle for the patient.

This innovative technique using BioCartilage to address OCD lesions of the capitellum shows promising results as reported in this subset of patients. Safe return to play is among the primary goals for patients who are frequently affected by this condition, and is directly impacted by the degree of invasive techniques used to address the lesion and the rehabilitation protocol postoperatively. This technique offers advantages by providing comparable, if not improved, range of motion as compared to current techniques, with minimal complications and relatively rapid, safe return to sport with restoration of full, painless range of motion.

5 Editors View

This technique is another way to improve outcomes using biology. OCD lesions of the capitellum can be difficult to treat and the goal is to improve the healing capacity as much as possible. We feel this technique accomplishes that goal with the use of PRP and BioCartilage.

References

1. Smith MV, Bedi A, Chen NC. Surgical treatment for osteochondritis dissecans of the capitellum. Sports Health. 2012;4(5):425–32. https://doi.org/10.1177/1941738112444707.
2. Churchill RW, Munoz J, Ahmad CS. Osteochondritis dissecans of the elbow. Curr Rev Musculoskelet Med. 2016;9(2):232–9. https://doi.org/10.1007/s12178-016-9342-y.
3. Caldwell PE 3rd, Auerbach B, Pearson SE. Arthroscopic treatment of capitellum osteochondritis dissecans with micronized allogeneic cartilage scaffold. Arthrosc Tech. 2017;6(3):e815–20. Published 2017 Jun 19. https://doi.org/10.1016/j.eats.2017.04.007.
4. Fortier LA, Chapman HS, Pownder SL, Roller BL, Cross JA, Cook JL, Cole BJ. BioCartilage improves cartilage repair compared with microfracture alone in an equine model of full-thickness cartilage loss. Am J Sports Med. 2016;44(9):2366–74. https://doi.org/10.1177/0363546516648644. Epub 2016 Jun 13
5. Shimozono Y, Huang H, Deyer T, Kennedy JG. Comparison of functional and MRI outcomes of microfracture with and without BioCartilage for osteochondral lesions of the talus. Foot & Ankle Orthop. 2019; https://doi.org/10.1177/2473011419S00389.
6. Brusalis CM, Greditzer HG 4th, Fabricant PD, Stannard JP, Cook JL. BioCartilage augmentation of marrow stimulation procedures for cartilage defects of the knee: two-year clinical outcomes. Knee. 2020;27(5):1418–25. https://doi.org/10.1016/j.knee.2020.07.087.
7. Takahara M, Ogino T, Sasaki I, Kato H, Minami A, Kaneda K. Long term outcome of osteochondritis dissecans of the humeral capitellum. Clin Orthop Relat Res. 1999;363:108–15.
8. Vogt S, Siebenlist S, Hensler D, et al. Osteochondral transplantation in the elbow leads to good clinical and radiologic long-term results: an 8- to 14-year follow-up examination. Am J Sports Med. 2011;39(12):2619–25. https://doi.org/10.1177/0363546511420127.

Part II

Minimally Invasive Nanoarthroscopy

The History of Arthroscopy

Shane Taylor and Charles Giangarra

Arthroscopy has been a monumental change to the approach of joint ailments. It has a high degree of accuracy as it provides direct visualization of pathology and allows for treatment of conditions with a low morbidity due to its minimally invasive approach [1]. While arthroscopy is seen as a more modern revelation and is a staple of the treatment of joint ailments, its history dates back to 1806 and it faced a significant amount of resistance in its beginning stages [2]. Bozzini (1773–1809) developed the "Lichtleiter," which is the first known instrument to look into the bladder. He presented it to the Rome Academy of Science in 1806, but it was deemed only to be an instrument of interest [2]. Approximately 50 years later Desormaux was credited with the beginning of endoscopy with his "gazogene cystoscope." Instrumentation was able to develop further in 1879 when Edison developed the incandescent light bulb which allowed for a source of light that could be implemented into instruments to light body cavities [2].

The term arthroscopy was first used by Dr. Severin Nordentoft (1866–1922) in a manuscript which he published following his presentation to the 41st Congress of the German Society of Surgeons in 1912. However, Dr. Kenji Takagi (1888–1963) from Tokyo is the first true developer of arthroscopy and is given credit as the first to apply the principles of endoscopy to the knee joint (Fig. 1). In 1931, he developed the first practical arthroscope. It was 3.5 mm in diameter and was also the first mention of using saline to distend the knee joint. The Second World War slowed down advancements in arthroscopy, but following the war, Dr. Masaki Watanabe (1921–1994) who was mentored by Dr. Kenji Takagi developed the number 14 arthroscope which introduced a second portal for a light source and he was able to

S. Taylor (✉)
PGY1 Marshall University, Scott Depot, WV, USA
e-mail: taylorsh@marshall.edu

C. Giangarra
Department of Orthopaedic Surgery, VA Medical Center, Marshall University, Marshall University School of Medicine, Scott Depot, WV, USA

C. Lavender (ed.), *Biologic and Nanoarthroscopic Approaches in Sports Medicine*, https://doi.org/10.1007/978-3-030-71323-2_11

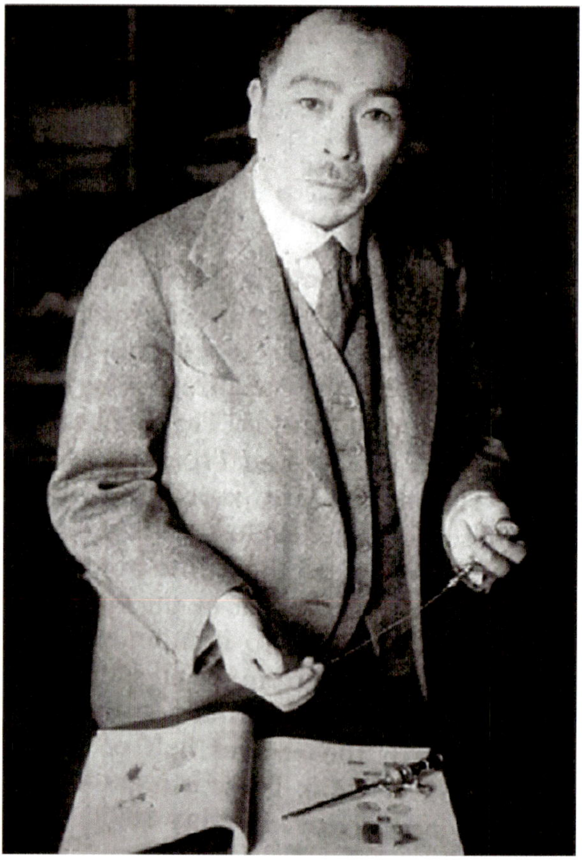

Fig. 1 Dr. Kenji Takagi

take the first color photographs of the inside of the knee. It was not until the 21st arthroscope that he developed the first production arthroscope (Fig. 2). This scope had a 101° of view and was also the last to use the incandescent light bulb as it was the number 22 arthroscope that used the fiber as its light source [2]. Dr. Watanabe had many other "firsts" in his career. He implemented the technique of triangulation and did the first procedure purely under arthroscopic control, removing a giant cell tumor, as well as the first partial meniscectomy [2] which is now the most commonly performed orthopedic procedure in the United States [3]. Dr. Robert W Jackson (1932–2010) was among the first to push the use of arthroscopy in North America. He twice went to visit and learn from Dr. Watanabe. He arranged the first arthroscopy learning labs and published the first textbook in English on Arthroscopy [2] (Fig. 3).

Another major advancement came with the invention of television and cameras that were small enough to be placed in an arthroscope. This allowed for everyone in the operating room to see what was being done on the screen. It also allowed for the surgeon to see inside the joint without the use of an eyepiece which was a potential source of contamination of the surgical field [1]. As there were

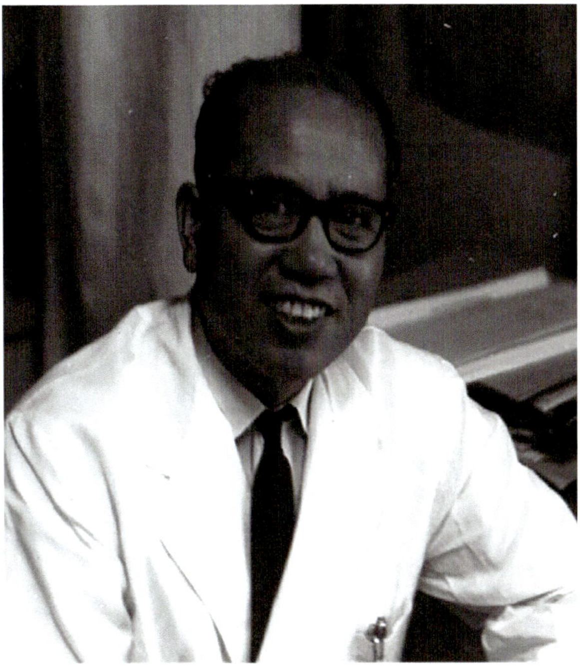

Fig. 2 Dr. Masaki Watanabe

advancements in the technology of the arthroscope that allowed them to be smaller, more functional, and with better visualization, there were advancements in other instruments that could be introduced into the joint to allow for procedures to be performed under arthroscopic guidance. Dr. T Whipple developed the suction punch. Drs. O'Connor, Dandy, and Jackson developed graspers and cutting tools. Dr. Lanny Johnson led to the development of many devices, but most notable was the motorized suction shaver and the "golden retriever" [4]. As the arthroscope and instrumentation improved, techniques developed rapidly to perform more procedures using arthroscopy including meniscus repairs and transplantations. Most of these developments up to now have been in reference to its use in the knee joint, but techniques were developed to apply arthroscopy to the shoulder, elbow, and ankle. Arthroscopy has continued to expand and be applied to wrist and hip pathologies [4].

As mentioned previously, these advancements in arthroscopy were not always smooth or greeted with enthusiasm. Dr. Phillip Heinrich Kreuscher (1883–1943) wrote a letter saying that at one point he stopped using an arthroscope because he did not find a case in which it was definitively indicated and he had frustrations with the imperfect technology. Dr. Michael Burman (1896–1974) had enough material for an Atlas of Arthroscopy, but it was not published because at the time its significance was not appreciated. Dr. Watanabe produced a colored video and showed it across the world with very little positive response [2]. It took time, persistence, and a lot of work from many individuals to prove the worth and benefits of arthroscopy.

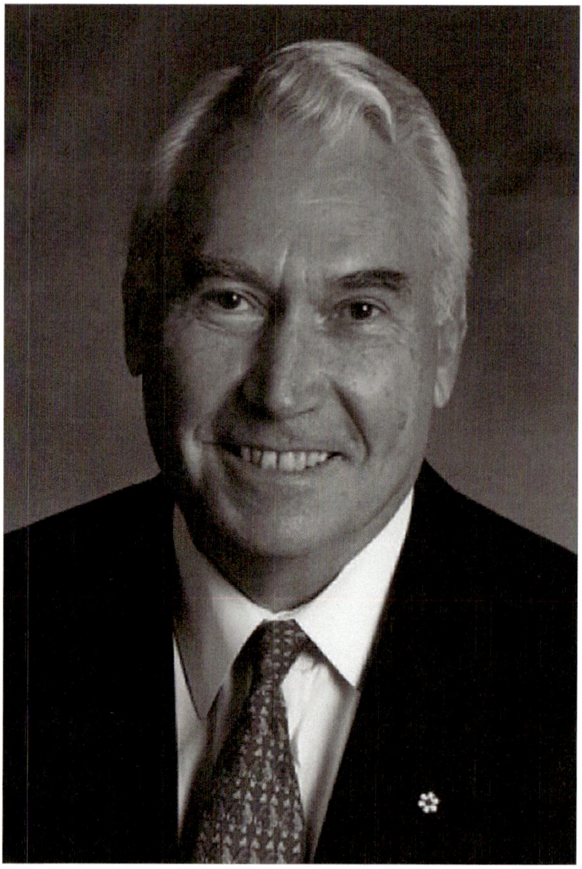

Fig. 3 Dr. Robert W Jackson

Today the arthroscope is advancing to nano-arthroscopy. Biomet released the InnerVue scope in 2005. This was a disposable arthroscope with an outer diameter of 1.2 mm with the goal of allowing physicians to view the joint in the office under local anesthesia. This would allow the physician and patient to visualize the pathology in the office and discuss treatment options. However, this scope was purely designed for diagnostic purposes, and if the patient elected, there would still be a need to schedule surgery and perform the procedure using normal instrumentation. The NanoScope from Arthrex is 1.9 mm in diameter with a 2.2 mm inflow sheath. It allows for visualization on 4 K screens with 400 × 400 resolution with a 120° field of view. The NanoScope with its associated nano-sized instruments allow the physician to perform operations using this smaller scope and have allowed for single incision rotator cuff repairs and incisionless meniscectomies [5–7].

Arthroscopy may be the most important event in orthopedics and it is fascinating to see how the treatment of joint pathology has moved from the large arthrotomies to, in some cases, incisionless scopes. Arthroscopy has allowed for increased diagnostic accuracy, less invasive surgery, decreased morbidity, and faster recoveries. Arthroscopy will continue to be a mainstay of orthopedic treatment of joint pathologies and an essential skill for an orthopedic surgeon.

References

1. Phillips BB. General principles of arthroscopy. In: Azar FM, Beaty JH, Canale ST, editors. Campbell's operative orthopedics. Philadelphia: Elsevier; 2017. p. 2458–9.
2. Jackson RW. A history of arthroscopy. Arthroscopy. 2010;26:92–103.
3. Lavender C, Lycans D, SAS A, Kopiec A, Schmicker T. Incisionless partial medial meniscectomy. Arthrosc Tech. 2020;9:375–8.
4. Jackson RW. History of arthroscopy. In: Andrews JR, Timmerman LA, editors. Diagnostic and operative arthroscopy. Philadelphia: W.B Saunders Company; 1997. p. 3–5.
5. InnerVue Diagnostic Scope System. Arthrotek. 2005. http://www.biomet.co.uk/resource/2019/Innervue%20Brochure.pdf.
6. NanoScope Nano Operative Arthroscopy System. Arthrex. 2019. https://www.arthrex.com/resources/brochures/OccqLfeqE0WWgQFr16DPfQ/nanoscope-nano-operative-arthroscopy-system. Accessed 9/29/2020.
7. Lavender C, Lycans D, SAS A, Berdis G. Single-incision rotator cuff repair with a needle arthroscope. Arthrosc Tech. 2020;9:419–23.

Introduction to Nanoarthroscopy

Dana Lycans and Chad Lavender

1 Introduction

The advent of arthroscopy within the field of orthopedic surgery has ushered in a new era where large incisions are rarely used anymore. This game-changing technology has changed how the surgery is performed altogether and has led to a better understanding of anatomy and pathology. Despite advances in imaging modalities, arthroscopy remains the gold standard in diagnosing intra-articular pathology. This is most commonly performed on the shoulder, elbow, wrist, knee, and ankle. Over the past decade, hip arthroscopy has emerged as a common surgery. Again, this has led to an increased understanding of joint anatomy as well as pathologic processes that has proven to be beneficial to many patients.

The days of large incisions, complex approaches, and the morbidity associated with these are long gone with most surgeons getting significant training in arthroscopic procedures. Now, rotator cuff repairs, anterior cruciate ligament reconstructions, labral repairs in the hip and shoulder, osteochondroplasties, meniscectomies, microfractures, and more can all be achieved through incisions less than 1 cm in length. This has improved patient outcomes and sped up patient recovery time. It is believed that decreased recovery time may be attributed to less invasive instrumentation as well as less arthroscopy fluid introduced into the joint.

D. Lycans (✉)
Sports Medicine Division, Department of Orthopaedic Surgery, Marshall University School of Medicine, Huntington, West Virginia, USA
e-mail: lycans@marshall.edu

C. Lavender
Orthopaedic Surgery Sports Medicine, Marshall University, Scott Depot, WV, USA

C. Lavender (ed.), *Biologic and Nanoarthroscopic Approaches in Sports Medicine*, https://doi.org/10.1007/978-3-030-71323-2_12

2 History

The concept of needle arthroscopy has been around for over 25 years. Ostendorf et al. used miniarthroscopy with 1–1.9 mm arthroscopes to help diagnose rheumatoid arthritis in a cadaveric study [1]. This was found to allow for the grading of synovial alterations, chondromalacia, and bony alterations. Synovial biopsies were also performed to help stage the disease in the metacarpophalangeal joints. Using a two-portal technique, this allowed for visualization of about 80% of the joint surface thus giving wonderful insight into the disease. Later, this group found miniarthroscopy to correlate well with MRI findings associated with rheumatoid arthritis in a cohort of patients [2].

A study was undertaken in 1995 by Gramas et al. to evaluate the efficacy of needle arthroscopy, standard arthroscopy, physical examination, and magnetic resonance imaging (MRI) of chronic knee pain [3]. In this small study, nine adults were included. Each of these patients had failed routine nonoperative treatment modalities such as anti-inflammatories, physical therapy, and Tylenol. They were each suspected to have a meniscal tear or osteoarthritis. Six of these patients underwent MRI. Arthroscopy was performed first with a needle arthroscopy. The needle arthroscope was 1.6 mm in diameter (Citscope-16, Citation Medical Supplies, Reno, Nevada). Immediately following this, they were scoped with a 4.0 mm diameter Stryker arthroscope (Stryker, San Jose, California, a subdivision of Johnson and Johnson). No difference was found in the abilities to detect meniscal abnormalities between the needle and standard arthroscopes. The standard arthroscope did detect cartilage lesions in the medial and lateral compartments better than the needle arthroscope.

Much attention has been given to needle arthroscopy recently with a large surge in the literature after 2017. This is likely driven by the high cost of health care and magnetic resonance imaging. There is also a new push for in-office arthroscopy for the diagnosis and treatment of intra-articular pathology.

Several studies have evaluated the efficacy of needle arthroscopy and standard arthroscopy with magnetic resonance imaging. [4–9] These studies agree that diagnostic arthroscopy with either standard or needle arthroscopy can save money. One large, prospective blinded, multicenter trial performed by Gill et al. compared the accuracy and safety of diagnostic arthroscopy with MRI. The study enrolled 110 patients who underwent MRI, diagnostic arthroscopy using a VisionScope needle arthroscope followed by a standard arthroscopy. Their results concluded that in-office diagnostic arthroscopy was statistically equivalent to standard surgical diagnostic arthroscopy. They determined that in-office diagnostic imaging provides a more accurate picture and assessment of intra-articular pathology in the knee as well.

In an effort to further improve cost and diagnostic accuracy, in-office needle arthroscopy has been further investigated. Zhang et al. provided a very good systematic review of indications for diagnostic in-office arthroscopy [10]. This review included 9 clinical studies and 2 cost analyses. The nine clinical studies demonstrated superior results with in-office needle arthroscopy compared to MRI regarding sensitivity, specificity, positive predictive value, and negative predictive value. Their cost analysis studies revealed lower costs of in-office needle arthroscopy when used in place of an MRI for diagnostic purposes.

In-office needle arthroscopy can also speed up the process of confirming and even treating a suspected diagnosis. This may lessen time out of work, which would lessen the financial impact of prolonged diagnostic dilemmas and scheduling of finite advanced imaging resources.

The concept of in-office surgical procedures can be daunting for many in terms of safety. One case series evaluated consecutive diagnostic needle arthroscopies in 13 independent institutions. Of the 1419 cases included in the analysis, no major complications (infection, chondral toxicity, need for urgent care, or emergency room treatment after the procedure) were reported by the authors. Vasovagal events were reported 1.9% of the time. Post-procedure pain was also reported, but in only 0.3% of cases. Of note, the authors did not use antibiotics prior to entry into the joint or after the procedure [11].

3 Indications

There is an ever-expanding list of indications for Nanoarthroscopy. First introduced as a diagnostic tool for small joints of the hand, this instrument's role has now expanded into the knee and shoulder. Needle arthroscopy can be used for strictly diagnostic purposes, but nanoarthroscopic instrumentation is also increasing to help treat intra-articular pathologies. Even tendoscopy has been introduced [12]. Several surgeons are now able to perform an essentially incisionless (in the traditional sense) partial meniscectomy for simple meniscus tears using only a needle arthroscope and nano-instrumentation as described by Lavender et al. [13].

The range of indications also includes loose body removal, synovial biopsy, glenoid labral repair, and rotator cuff repair [14, 15]. The Nanoscope can also be used as an adjunct scope to aid in simultaneous visualization of multiple compartments of a joint, potentially saving time in the OR. This can also save the patient an incision, thus virtually eliminating a possible infection site.

4 Instrumentation

Many companies have introduced needle arthroscopes and video equipment as outlined in the studies mentioned earlier in this chapter. The system used by the author is the Arthrex (Naples, FL) NanoScope™ Operative Arthroscopy System. This system uses a flexible 1.9 mm disposable camera as well as 2 mm resection tools and cannulas. These tools include nearly a full armamentarium of options including retractable probes, scissors, graspers, biters, and shavers. The clarity of image and flexibility with these instruments are what make the Nanoscope(Arthrex) so much more successful than those that came before.

Different set-ups are made possible by manufacturers. If being used in the operating room, the camera and sheath can be hooked up to a standard arthroscopic video monitor and pump system as would be used for routine arthroscopy. Alternatively, if being used in an office setting, one could connect a saline-filled syringe to the cannula and insert fluid as needed. In this setting, a smaller video screen is available for viewing the video.

When operating without a tourniquet, in-flow is important. Arthrex (Naples, FL) has recently introduced the high flow cannula, which allows increased inflow of fluid into the joint, thus increasing pressure and improving visualization. This specifically can help with the visualization of the back of the knee or the shoulder.

5 Future Directions

While this concept has been around for more than two decades, nanoarthroscopy is still in its infancy. There are still obstacles to overcome. The initial cost of the in-office set up can be prohibitive in smaller orthopedic offices. Billing and reimbursement for in-office procedures can be confusing. Certainly, help can be obtained from industry representatives with billing procedures and resources.

As technology advances, better instrumentation will undoubtedly arise. This will further increase the indications and efficacy of nanoarthroscopy bringing it more into the mainstream. With numerous cost-analysis studies being performed and confirming needle arthroscopy to be a cheaper route to diagnosis and treatment of pathology, this will likely gain popularity as a viable option to decrease healthcare costs. More studies and specifically randomized trials will need to be performed confirming the effectiveness of this intervention if it is to be accepted widely by the orthopedics community. With the rapidly expanding instrumentation and popularity of needle arthroscopy, these studies will soon follow.

References

1. Ostendorf B, Dann P, Wedekind F, et al. Miniarthroscopy of metacarpophalangeal joints in rheumatoid arthritis. Rating of diagnostic value in synovitis staging and efficiency of synovial biopsy. J Rheumatol. 1999;26(9):1901–8.
2. Ostendorf B, Peters R, Dann P, et al. Magnetic resonance imaging and miniarthroscopy of metacarpophalangeal joints: sensitive detection of morphologic changes in rheumatoid arthritis. Arthritis Rheum. 2001;44(11):2492–502. https://doi.org/10.1002/1529-0131(200111)44:11<2492::aid-art429>3.0.co;2-x.
3. Gramas DA, Antounian FS, Peterfy CG, Genant HK, Lane NE. Assessment of needle arthroscopy, standard arthroscopy, physical examination, and magnetic resonance imaging in knee pain: a pilot study. J Clin Rheumatol Pract Rep Rheum Musculoskelet Dis. 1995;1(1):26–34. https://doi.org/10.1097/00124743-199502000-00007.
4. Voigt JD, Mosier M, Huber B. Diagnostic needle arthroscopy and the economics of improved diagnostic accuracy: a cost analysis. Appl Health Econ Health Policy. 2014;12(5):523–35. https://doi.org/10.1007/s40258-014-0109-6.

5. Deirmengian CA, Dines JS, Vernace JV, Schwartz MS, Creighton RA, Gladstone JN. Use of a small-bore needle arthroscope to diagnose intra-articular knee pathology: comparison with magnetic resonance imaging. Am J Orthop Belle Mead NJ. 2018;47(2) https://doi.org/10.12788/ajo.2018.0007.
6. Amin N, McIntyre L, Carter T, Xerogeanes J, Voigt J. Cost-effectiveness analysis of needle arthroscopy versus magnetic resonance imaging in the diagnosis and treatment of meniscal tears of the knee. Arthrosc J Arthrosc Relat Surg Off Publ Arthrosc Assoc N Am Int Arthrosc Assoc. 2019;35(2):554–562.e13. https://doi.org/10.1016/j.arthro.2018.09.030.
7. Cooper DE. Editorial commentary: the desire to take a look: surgeons and patients must weigh the benefits and costs of in-office needle arthroscopy versus magnetic resonance imaging. Arthrosc J Arthrosc Relat Surg Off Publ Arthrosc Assoc N Am Int Arthrosc Assoc. 2018;34(8):2436–7. https://doi.org/10.1016/j.arthro.2018.06.002.
8. Gill TJ, Safran M, Mandelbaum B, Huber B, Gambardella R, Xerogeanes J. A prospective, blinded, multicenter clinical trial to compare the efficacy, accuracy, and safety of in-office diagnostic arthroscopy with magnetic resonance imaging and surgical diagnostic arthroscopy. Arthrosc J Arthrosc Relat Surg Off Publ Arthrosc Assoc N Am Int Arthrosc Assoc. 2018;34(8):2429–35. https://doi.org/10.1016/j.arthro.2018.03.010.
9. Voigt JD, Mosier M, Huber B. In-office diagnostic arthroscopy for knee and shoulder intra-articular injuries its potential impact on cost savings in the United States. BMC Health Serv Res. 2014;14:203. https://doi.org/10.1186/1472-6963-14-203.
10. Zhang K, Crum RJ, Samuelsson K, Cadet E, Ayeni OR, de Sa D. In-office needle arthroscopy: a systematic review of indications and clinical utility. Arthrosc J Arthrosc Relat Surg Off Publ Arthrosc Assoc N Am Int Arthrosc Assoc. 2019;35(9):2709–21. https://doi.org/10.1016/j.arthro.2019.03.045.
11. McMillan S, Chhabra A, Hassebrock JD, Ford E, Amin NH. Risks and complications associated with intra-articular arthroscopy of the knee and shoulder in an office setting. Orthop J Sports Med. 2019;7(9):2325967119869846. https://doi.org/10.1177/2325967119869846.
12. Stornebrink T, Stufkens SAS, Appelt D, Wijdicks CA, Kerkhoffs GMMJ. 2-mm diameter operative tendoscopy of the tibialis posterior, peroneal, and achilles tendons: a cadaveric study. Foot Ankle Int. 2020;41(4):473–8. https://doi.org/10.1177/1071100719895504.
13. Lavender C, Lycans D, Sina Adil SA, Kopiec A, Schmicker T. Incisionless partial medial meniscectomy. Arthrosc Tech. 2020;9(3):e375–8. https://doi.org/10.1016/j.eats.2019.11.003.
14. Lavender C, Lycans D, Kopiec A, Sayan A. Nanoscopic single-incision anterior labrum repair. Arthrosc Tech. 2020;9(3):e297–301. https://doi.org/10.1016/j.eats.2019.10.010.
15. Lavender C, Lycans D, Sina Adil SA, Berdis G. Single-incision rotator cuff repair with a needle arthroscope. Arthrosc Tech. 2020;9(4):e419–23. https://doi.org/10.1016/j.eats.2019.11.012.

Incisionless Partial Medial Meniscectomy

Andrew Fontaine and Chad Lavender

1 Introduction

Minimally invasive surgery results in reduced pain, swelling, complications, and a quicker recovery. Arthroscopic knee surgery has evolved greatly from its inception in the twentieth century. Arthroscopic meniscectomy is the most commonly performed orthopedic surgical procedure in the United States. Kim et al. [1] showed that the number of arthroscopic partial meniscectomies increased by 49% to approximately 500,000 between 1996 and 2006 in the United States. The diagnosis of intra-articular pathology such as meniscal tears depends on history, physical examination, and imaging modalities including plain radiography and magnetic resonance imaging (MRI). Arthroscopy is the gold standard in diagnosis because it allows direct visualization of pathology. MRI, although incredibly valuable, is not perfect; in a recent meta-analysis. Phelan et al. [2] evaluated the diagnostic accuracy of MRI in knee pathology specifically anterior cruciate ligament tears and meniscal injuries. The authors found that for anterior cruciate ligament tears, the sensitivity and specificity of MRI were 87% and 93%, for medial meniscal tears 89% and 88%, respectively, and for lateral meniscal tears 78% and 95%, respectively. Although Phelan et al. [2] found compelling numbers for the diagnostic accuracy using MRI, this modality can be an expensive proposition, and with the rising cost of health care, it

With Permission Arthroscopy Techniques Chad Lavender, M.D., Dana Lycans, M.D., Syed Ali Sina Adil, M.D., Adam Kopiec, M.D.,Thomas Schmicker, M.D. Incisionless Partial Medial Meniscectomy: *Arthroscopy Techniques* 2020;9 pp e 375–378.

A. Fontaine
PGY4 Marshall University, Huntington, WV, USA

C. Lavender (✉)
Orthopaedic Surgery Sports Medicine, Marshall University, Scott Depot, WV, USA

C. Lavender (ed.), *Biologic and Nanoarthroscopic Approaches in Sports Medicine*, https://doi.org/10.1007/978-3-030-71323-2_13

calls into question whether there is a better, more cost-effective way to evaluate joint pathology.

The NanoScope needle arthroscopy system (Arthrex, Naples, FL) is both diagnostic and therapeutic in that it allows direct visualization of intra-articular pathology and for instrumentation to treat meniscal tears. Although needle arthroscopy is mainly studied as a diagnostic tool that may be used in an in-office setting, the capabilities of the NanoScope system allow it to become a substitute for regular arthroscopy in certain cases such as partial meniscectomies as demonstrated in this technique. The NanoScope eliminates the need for incisions, requiring only a spinal needle to establish access to the joint.

2 Indications

This technique can be used in any patient with a standard meniscus tear in which you would consider arthroscopy.

3 Contraindications

Complex meniscus tears which may require more resection, however this can be decided intraoperatively. Large patients where anatomic landmarks are difficult to palpate.

4 Surgical Technique

4.1 Patient Setup

The patient is placed in the supine position with the operative extremity in a leg holder and a tourniquet applied to the operative thigh. The nonoperative extremity is placed over a well-padded pillow in slight flexion. The operative extremity is exsanguinated, and the tourniquet is inflated.

4.2 NanoScope Insertion

A spinal needle is inserted into anterolateral joint space while the knee is in full extension (Fig. 1). A nitinol wire is inserted into the needle, and the needle is removed. A small cannula is then inserted over the wire and the wire is removed. Inflow is then placed onto the cannula, and the NanoScope is inserted for visualization of the joint. A standard diagnostic arthroscopy is then performed in the patellofemoral joint. The NanoScope is then redirected into the medial joint space.

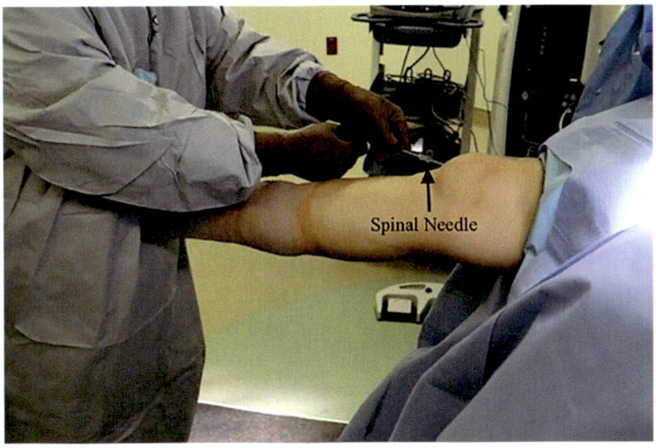

Fig. 1 Viewing the right knee from outside of the knee, the spinal needle is seen inserted into the patellofemoral joint while the knee is in full extension

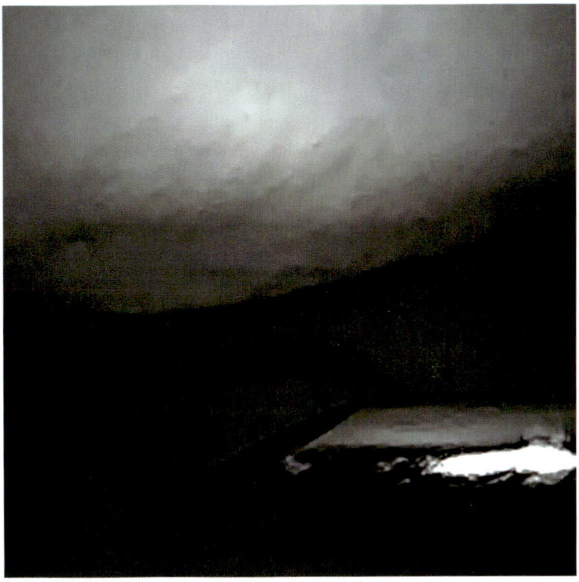

Fig. 2 Viewing the medial joint space with the 0° NanoScope while the right knee is in flexion, a spinal needle is seen inserted into the medial joint space

4.3 Medial Portal

An 18-gauge spinal needle is then used to localize the medial portal location in an outside fashion (Fig. 2). A nitinol wire is inserted into the needle and the needle is removed (Fig. 3). A small 2.7-mm cannula is then inserted over the wire, and the wire is removed.

4.4 Partial Medial Meniscectomuy

Nano Instruments (Arthrex) are then used through this medial portal to perform the partial medial meniscectomy (Figs. 4, 5, and 6). First, the NanoBiter (Arthrex) is

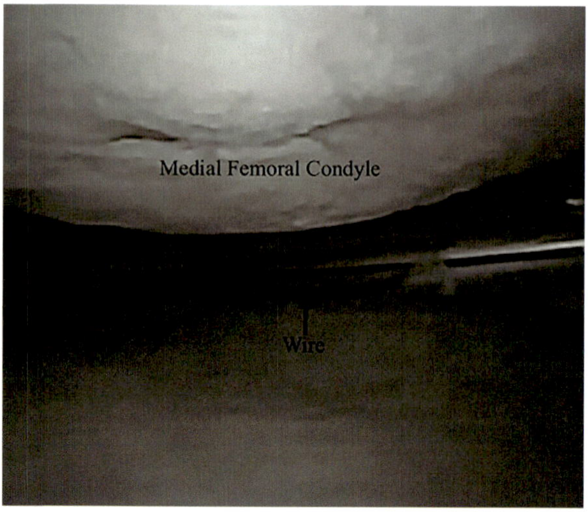

Fig. 3 Viewing the medial joint space with the 0° NanoScope while the right knee is in flexion, a spinal needle is seen inserted into the medial joint space. A nitinol wire has been placed through the spinal needle

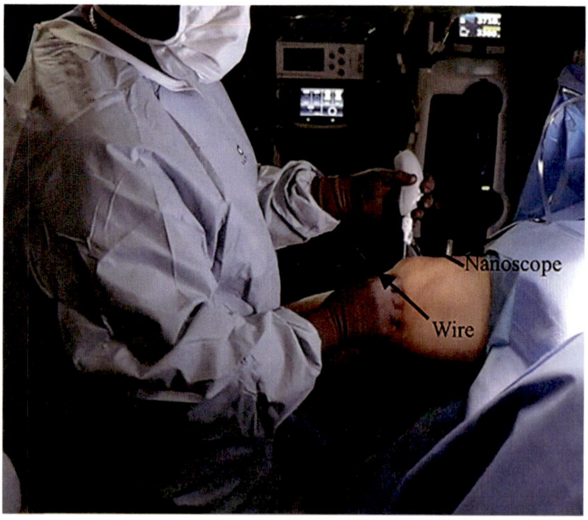

Fig. 4 Viewing the right knee from outside of the joint, the NanoScope is seen placed through the lateral joint space, and the spinal needle can be seen in the medial joint space

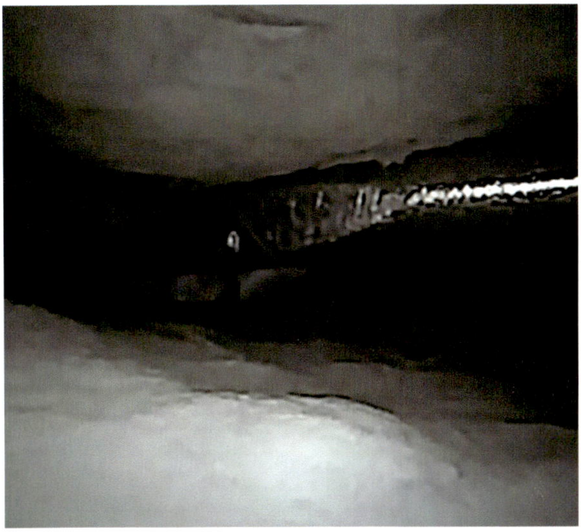

Fig. 5 Viewing the medial joint space with the 0° NanoScope while the right knee is in flexion, a nanobiter is seen performing the first steps of the partial medial meniscectomy

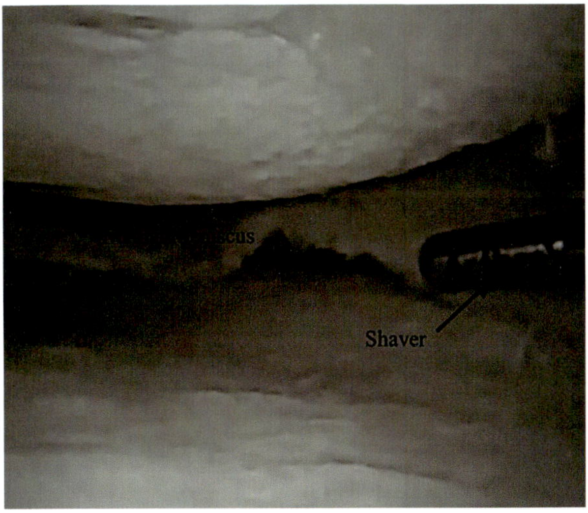

Fig. 6 Viewing the medial joint space with the 0° NanoScope while the right knee is in flexion, a nanoshaver is seen finishing the partial medial meniscectomy

used to bite the posterior horn of the medial meniscus. A small Nano Shaver (Arthrex) is then used to finish the meniscectomy (Figs. 7 and 8). Alternatively, it may be helpful to remove the small cannula and percutaneously place a 3-mm shaver, which will allow more aggressive shaving. A view from outside the joint is shown revealing no obvious incisions (Fig. 9).

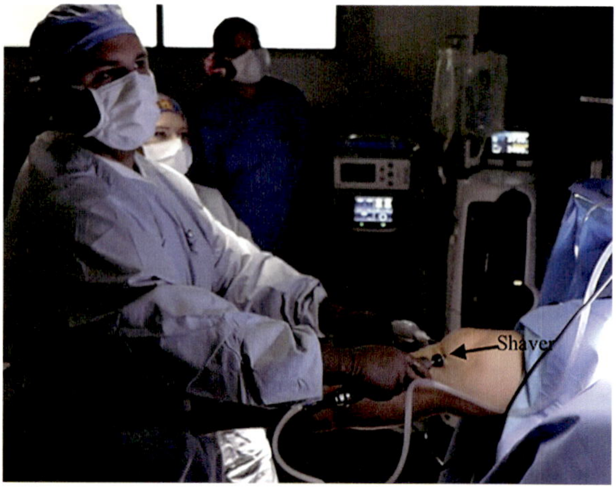

Fig. 7 Viewing the right knee from outside the joint, the NanoScope can be seen in the lateral joint space, and nanoshaver can be seen performing the partial medial meniscectomy

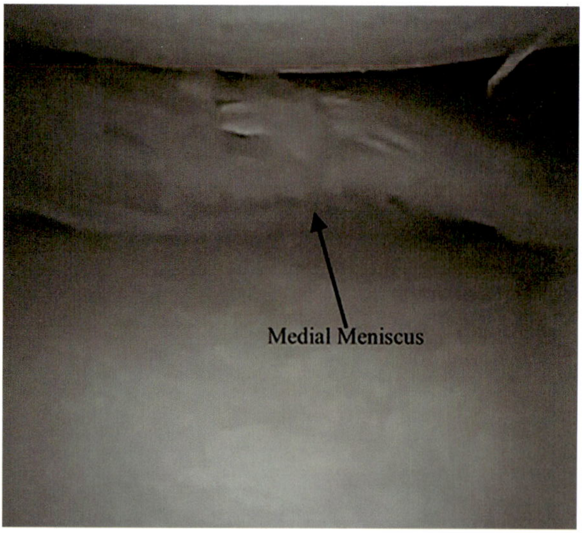

Fig. 8 Viewing the medial joint space with the 0° NanoScope while the right knee is in flexion, the final partial medial meniscectomy has been performed

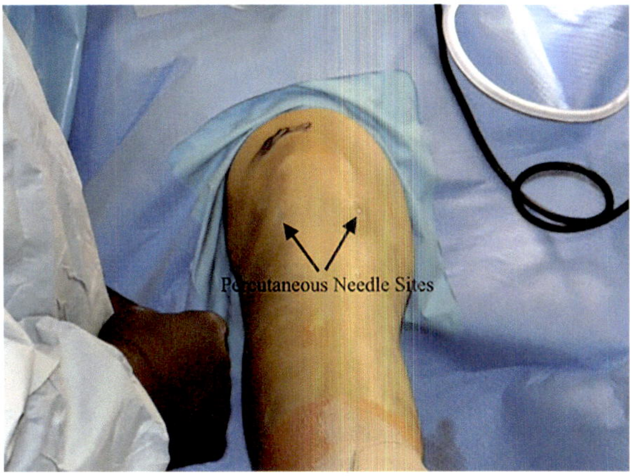

Fig. 9 Viewing the right knee from outside the joint shows percutaneous needle sites but no incisions

5 Discussion

Needle arthroscopy in the form of the NanoScope promises to be a minimally invasive method for diagnosis and treatment of intra-articular pathology. Currently, most data on needle arthroscopy compare the advantages it provides in an in-office setting for diagnostic purposes of intra-articular pathology in comparison with MRI. Gill et al. compared VisionScope needle arthroscopy to MRI and surgical diagnostic arthroscopy in 110 patients and found no statistically significant difference regarding the diagnosis of intra-articular, non-ligamentous knee joint pathology [3]. These results were also found in a similar study by Xerogeanes et al. [4] where they showed that needle arthroscopy is more accurate than MRI and statistically equivalent to surgical arthroscopy. Deirmengian et al. [5] also conducted a study where they evaluated the use of needle arthroscopy compared with MRI for the diagnosis of knee pathology. They found needle arthroscopy to be superior to MRI in both sensitivity and specificity in diagnosing meniscal tears (92.6% vs 77.8%; 100% vs 41.7%, respectively) and articular cartilage pathology. This incisionless technique presented in this chapter was originally published by Lavender [6].

The incisionless partial medial meniscectomy technique focuses on the treatment of pathology using a NanoScope in addition to the diagnostic purpose. There are several pearls mentioned above included redirecting the Nanoscope gently into each compartment and using a 3mm shaver percutaneously (Table 1). This technique allows the surgeon a minimally invasive approach with the full capability of regular arthroscopy when treating partial meniscal tears. With this technique there are several advantages including there is no need to make an incision (Table 2). A portal is made with a 2.7-mm cannula, requiring only a spinal needle to establish access. The technique described here can also be translated into an office-based setting without

Table 1 Pearls and pitfalls of the incisionless partial medial meniscectomy

Pearls
The medial cannula can be removed and a 3-mm shaver inserted percutaneously for more aggressive shaving
The NanoScope should be redirected into compartments for each new viewing angle
Pitfalls
Care should be taken not to be overly aggressive with the small instruments

Table 2 Advantages and disadvantages of the incisionless partial medial meniscectomy

Advantages
Decreased loss and need for fluid
Less swelling and pain
Decreased risk for wound infection
Disadvantages
Additional cost of NanoScope
Difficult viewing angles

Table 3 Risk and limitations of incisionless partial medial meniscectomy

Risks
Quality of image is slightly lower, which may lead to missed secondary diagnosis
Larger meniscus tears may be more difficult to manage with smaller instruments
Instruments are smaller and more fragile

the need for general anesthesia. There are limitations to the NanoScope because it has a lower image quality than most standard arthroscopes (Table 3). This could limit the identification of secondary diagnoses and conditions. This procedure is also limited to smaller meniscus tears because larger tears may be difficult to manage without more flow or larger shavers (Table 2). As surgery heads more and more toward minimally invasive and cost-effective procedures; techniques such as the one we present here could lead to improved outcomes for patients.

6 Editor's View

This technique is one of our first truly incisionless techniques. The fact that we can do a partial meniscectomy without making an incision is a remarkable step forward in arthroscopy. Obviously not making an incision and performing the procedure percutaneously decreases the risk to the patient and also should improve our early outcomes. Patients that have had this procedure have walked out of the hospital with very minimal complaints of pain and I think can return earlier to sport and activity. One question I have been asked is what defines an incisionless procedure and in my opinion if you do not need to use a knife to make an incision we consider that percutaneous as this technique shows. I look forward to seeing further innovation in multiple joints focusing on incisionless procedures such as this partial meniscectomy.

References

1. Kim S, Bosque J, Meehan JP, Jamali A, Marder R. Increase in outpatient knee arthroscopy in the United States: a comparison of national surveys of ambulatory surgery, 1996 and 2006. J Bone Joint Surg Am. 2011;93:994–1000.
2. Phelan N, Rowland P, Galvin R, O'Byrne JM. A systematic review and meta-analysis of the diagnostic accuracy of MRI for suspected ACL and meniscal tears of the knee. Knee Surg Sports Traumatol Arthrosc. 2016;24:1525–39.
3. Gill TJ, Safran M, Mandelbaum B, Huber B, Gambardella R, Xerogeanes J. A prospective, blinded, multicenter clinical trial to compare the efficacy, accuracy, and safety of in-office diagnostic arthroscopy with magnetic resonance imaging and surgical diagnostic arthroscopy. Arthroscopy. 2018;34:2429–35.
4. Xerogeanes JW, Safran MR, Huber B, Mandelbaum BR, Robertson W, Gambardella RA. A prospective multi-center clinical trial to compare efficiency, accuracy and safety of the VisionScope imaging system compared to MRI and diagnostic arthroscopy. Orthop J Sports Med. 2014;2(Suppl2):2325967114.
5. Deirmengian CA, Dines JS, Vernace JV, Schwartz MS, Creighton RA, Gladstone JN. Use of a small-bore needle arthroscope to diagnose intra-articular knee pathology: comparison with magnetic resonance imaging. Am J Orthop. 2018;47:1–5.
6. Lavender C, Lycans D, Adil SAS, Kopiec A, Schmicker T. Incisionless partial medial meniscectomy. Arthrosc Tech. 2020;9:e 375–8.

Nanoscopic Single-Incision Anterior Labrum Repair

Andrew Fontaine and Dana Lycans

1 Introduction

Anterior shoulder instability is a common problem affecting 1–2% of the general population. This number increases up to 15% for athletes participating in contact sports [1, 2]. Traditionally, open repair of a torn labrum has provided excellent results with high patient satisfaction scores and low reoperation rates [3–5]. This surgery, however, can be associated with a high morbidity and a significant loss of shoulder motion [5]. Arthroscopic Bankart repair, originally described by Wolf et al., has gained popularity as a less-invasive surgery that has been shown to provide equivalent results compared with open surgery [6, 7]. This is traditionally done with the use of a viewing portal in the back of the shoulder and 2 anterior working portals in the front of the shoulder.

A more minimally invasive approach using a single anterior working portal recently has been adopted by many surgeons. This also can be associated with lower patient morbidity [3, 8–10]. In sports medicine, we continue to try to provide improved outcomes by decreasing size and number of incisions, and in this technique, we describe a single-incision anterior labrum repair without the need for a posterior incision. Our technique uses the NanoScope (Arthrex, Naples, FL) to eliminate the posterior portal, achieving a single-incision arthroscopic anterior labrum repair.

With permission from Arthroscopy Techniques: Lavender, C, Lycans D, Kopiec, A, Sayan, A. Nanoscopic single-incision anterior labrum repair. *Arthrosc Tech*, 2020, 9:e297-e301.

A. Fontaine (✉)
PGY4 Marshall University, Huntington, WV, USA

D. Lycans
Sports Medicine Division, Department of Orthopaedic Surgery, Marshall University School of Medicine, Huntington, West Virginia, USA

C. Lavender (ed.), *Biologic and Nanoarthroscopic Approaches in Sports Medicine*, https://doi.org/10.1007/978-3-030-71323-2_14

2 Indications

Indications include anterior shoulder instability with standard Bankart labrum tears anteriorly with displacement. Patients who are unstable in need of a capsular shift also would be indicated for this procedure. Patients which have coagulopathies when you want to avoid bleeding as much as possible would be great candidates for this procedure.

3 Contraindications

Patients with large 360 type tears which need posterior work may need converted to a standard scope.

4 Surgical Technique

4.1 Patient Setup

The patient is placed in the lateral position with the operative extremity placed in a standard lateral arm positioner. An axillary roll is placed under the nonoperative extremity. The operative shoulder landmarks are marked out including the scapula, coracoid, and acromioclavicular joint.

4.2 Nanoscope Insertion

A spinal needle is inserted into the glenohumeral joint posteriorly (Fig. 1). In total, 30 cc of normal saline can be loaded into the joint to help with initial visualization. A nitinol wire is inserted into the needle and the needle is removed. A small 2.7-mm cannula is then inserted over the wire and the wire is removed (Fig. 2). Inflow is then placed onto the cannula and the NanoScope is inserted for visualization of the joint. A standard diagnostic arthroscopy is then performed identifying the anterior labrum tear.

4.3 Anterior Portal

An 18-gauge spinal needle is then used to localize the anterior portal location in an outside fashion (Fig. 3). A small incision is made and a switching stick is placed into the glenohumeral joint from anteriorly. An 8-mm dilator is then used to dilate for cannula insertion. The 8.25-mm cannula (Arthrex) is then placed into the joint from anteriorly for a working portal. Inflow is then switched to the anterior portal.

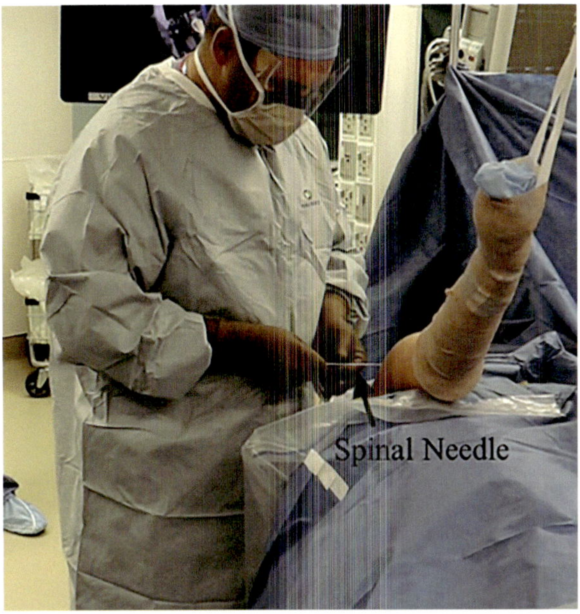

Fig. 1 Viewing the right shoulder in the lateral position, a spinal needle is inserted posteriorly

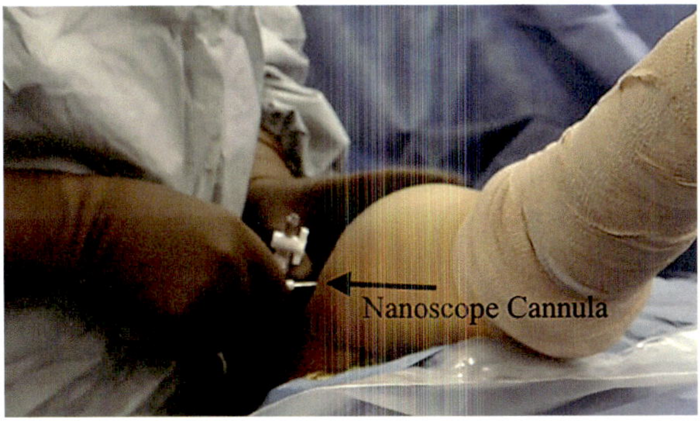

Fig. 2 Viewing the right shoulder from outside the joint, a 2.7 mm cannula is inserted posteriorly, over a nitinol wire

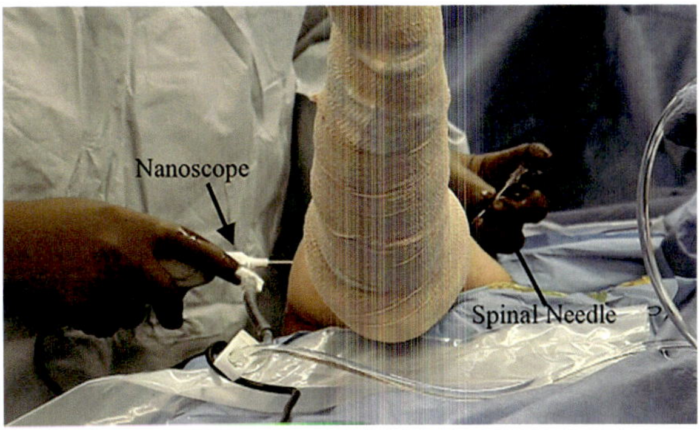

Fig. 3 Viewing the right shoulder from outside the joint, a spinal needle has been inserted anteriorly and the NanoScope (Arthrex) is placed through the posterior cannula

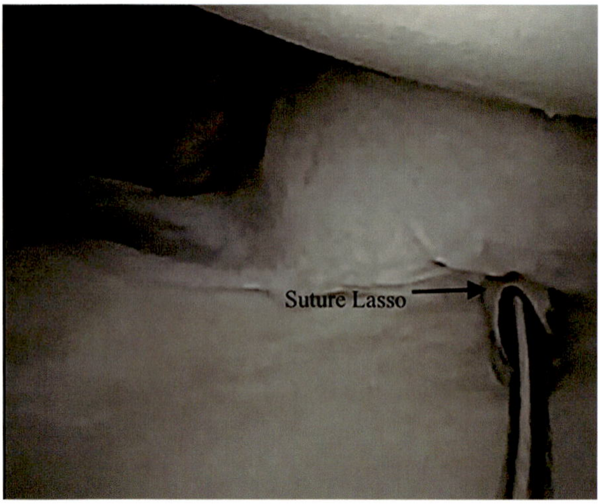

Fig. 4 Viewing the right shoulder posteriorly using the 0° NanoScope, the 45° suture lasso has been used to place a nitinol wire through the labrum

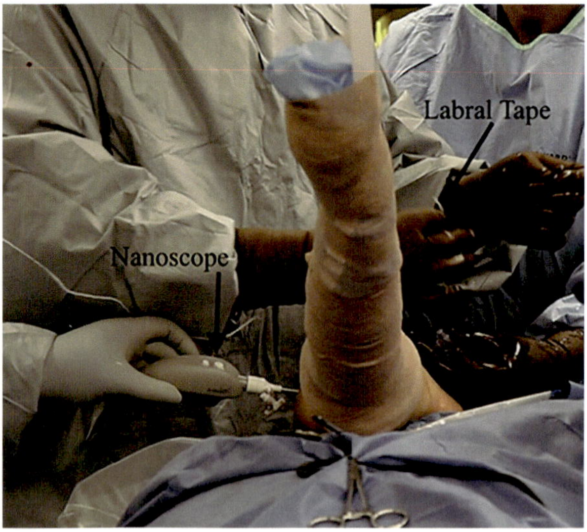

Fig. 5 Viewing the right shoulder from outside the joint, the nitinol wire is being pulled out of the anterior portal, loading the labral tape through the anterior labrum. The NanoScope is used to view from posteriorly

4.4 Labrum Repair

A small elevator and rasp are used to prepare the glenoid and labrum tear. A 45° to the right suture lasso is used to pass a nitinol wire loop through the anterior inferior labrum and this wire is retrieved (Fig. 4). Labral tape is then passed using this loop and pulled through the anterior inferior labrum (Fig. 5). Using a drill guide and the drill for the 2.9-mm PushLock anchor (Arthrex), the anchor hole is drilled in the anterior surface of the glenoid. The labral tape has been placed through the PushLock (Arthrex) anchor and tensioned as the PushLock is inserted into the glenoid (Fig. 6).

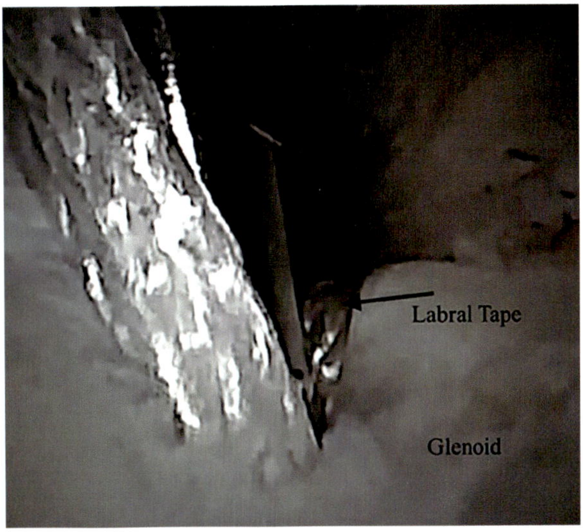

Fig. 6 Viewing the right shoulder posteriorly using the 0° NanoScope, a 2.9-mm PushLock anchor loaded with labral tape is seen being inserted through the glenoid

Table 1 Pearls and Pitfalls of the Single-Incision Anterior Labrum Repair

Pearls
Using the 30° arthroscope can aid in visualization anteriorly simultaneously
Inflow should be placed through the anterior working portal
Pitfalls
Improper placement of the posterior spinal needle can cause difficult visualization

At this point, the 30° arthroscope can be placed through the anterior portal for a view directly onto the labrum and we will view both angles simultaneously with the NanoScope (Arthrex) posteriorly (Table 1 and Fig. 7). These steps are repeated for 2 more superior anchors until the labrum is fully repaired and stable to probing (Fig. 8). At the end of the repair, we view from both portals simultaneously to give a view of the entire repair from various angles (Fig. 9).

5 Discussion

Arthroscopic anterior labral repair has grown significantly in popularity and is associated with less morbidity and equivalent outcomes when compared with open labral repair. We describe the use of the NanoScope to eliminate the posterior portal. This has many advantages [11]. First, it allows for the use of a single incision, leading to less morbidity for the patient and, theoretically, a lower surgical-site infection risk as there are fewer incisions (Fig. 10). Fewer holes created in the capsule mean

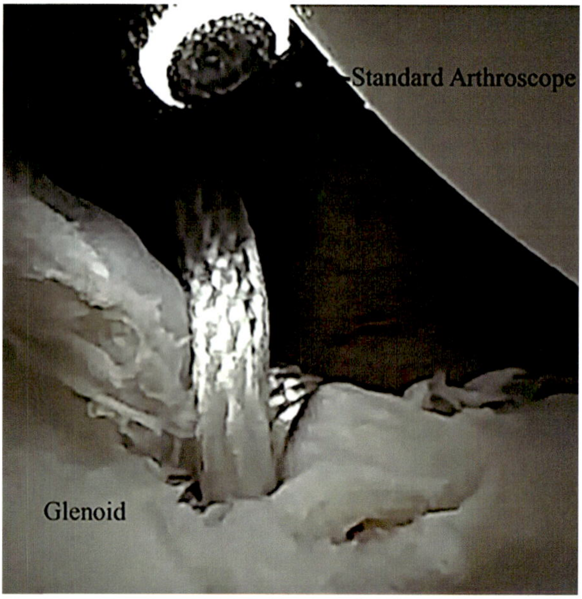

Fig. 7 Viewing the right shoulder posteriorly using the 0° NanoScope, the second anchor has been placed and you can see the 30° arthroscope has been placed into the anterior portal

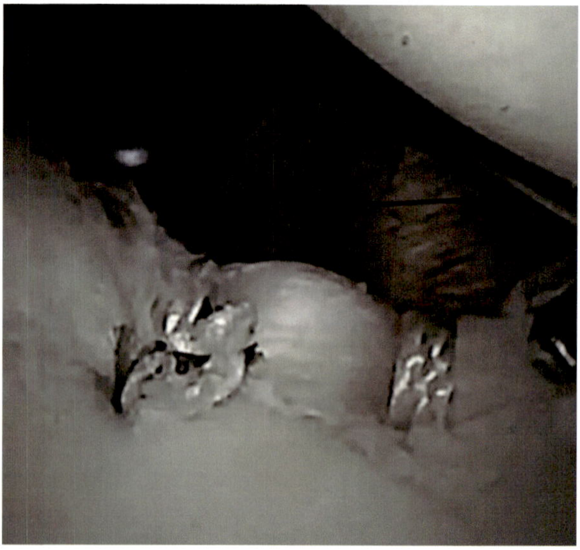

Fig. 8 Viewing the right shoulder posteriorly using the 0° NanoScope, you can see the final anterior labrum repair

less fluid extravasation to the surrounding soft tissues, leading to decreased swelling. This in turn may lead to less pain postoperatively. Because there is less extravasation of the arthroscopy fluid, it is easier to distend the shoulder for visualization and there is decreased need for fluid overall. Lastly, and most importantly, the 2.7-mm NanoScope inflow sheath causes less damage done to the posterior capsule and rotator cuff than the traditional 5.9-mm arthroscopic inflow sheath. This can then lead to an easier early recovery and return to function.

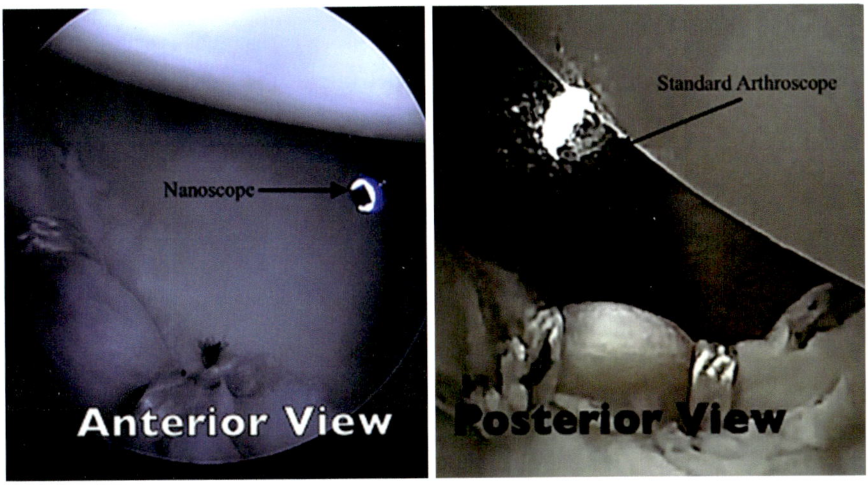

Fig. 9 The right side is a view of the right shoulder with the 0° NanoScope posteriorly. The left side is a view of the right shoulder with the 30° arthroscope from anteriorly

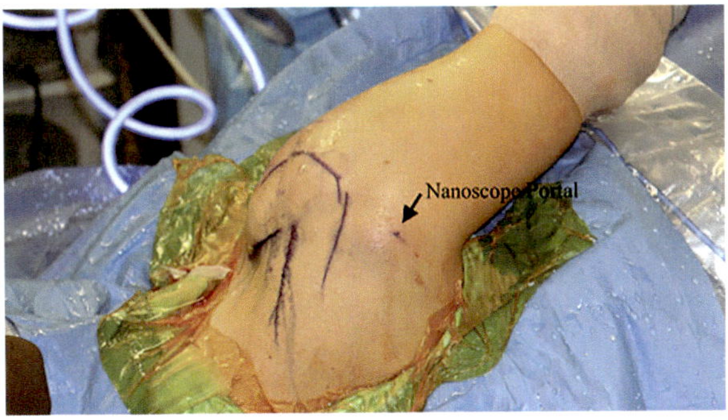

Fig. 10 View of the right shoulder from outside the joint in the lateral position, seeing there is no posterior incision

Table 2 Advantages and Disadvantages of the Single-Incision Anterior Labrum Repair

Advantages
Decreased loss and need for fluid
Less swelling and pain
Possible increase in motion
Disadvantages
Additional cost of NanoScope
Difficult viewing angles

Potential disadvantages of using this system include view limitations. Initial needle placement must be correct to allow for adequate visualization of the anterior labrum and capsular tissue (Table 2). The NanoScope is a 0-degree viewing camera, which can make it difficult to see down over the anterior rim of the glenoid from the posterior portal. This, however, can be overcome by inserting the traditional 4.0 mm 30° or 70° arthroscope through the anterior cannula giving a complete picture of the injury and repair. Because of these potential technical issues, one should never hesitate to abort and make a traditional posterior portal if the quality of the repair anteriorly is at risk.

We feel that the NanoScope (Arthrex) is a useful tool to decrease patient morbidity and possibly speed up recovery when used appropriately. Further studies are planned to evaluate subjective and objective outcomes in patients who have this surgery.

6 Editor's View

This technique really highlights the use of the nanoscope intra-articularly in the shoulder. One of the main advantages about this technique is that you can run your inflow through the anterior cannula providing nice distension of the glenohumeral joint and you can do a variety of procedures with only a percutaneous nanoscope portal posteriorly. We feel the overall outcome is less fluid used during surgery in addition to fewer portals for your labrum repair. Obviously, you could use the techniques described in this chapter and perform other procedures such as a biceps tenodesis, a debridement of the intra-articular space, a subscapularis repair, or other procedures inside the joint with just the nanoscope portal posteriorly. It will be interesting to see the results of a single incision labrum versus our standard arthroscopy labrum repairs.

References

1. Galvin JW, Ernat JJ, Waterman BR, Stadecker MJ, Parada SA. The epidemiology and natural history of anterior shoulder instability. Curr Rev Musculoskel Med. 2017;10:411–24.
2. Gottschalk LJ 4th, Walia P, Patel RM, et al. Stability of the glenohumeral joint with combined humeral head and glenoid defects: a cadaveric study. Am J Sports Med. 2016;44:933–40.
3. Ng DZ, Lau BPH, Tan BHM, Kumar VP. Single working portal technique for knotless arthroscopic Bankart repair. Arthrosc Tech. 2017;6:e1989–92.
4. Coughlin RP, Crapser A, Coughlin K, Coughlin LP. Open Bankart revisited. Arthrosc Tech. 2017;6:e233–7.
5. Khatri K, Arora H, Chaudhary S, Goyal D. Meta-analysis of randomized controlled trials involving anterior shoulder instability. Open Orthop J. 2018;12:411–8.
6. Huerta A, Rincón G, Peidro L, Combalia A, Sastre S. Controversies in the surgical management of shoulder instability: open vs arthroscopic procedures. Open Orthop J. 2017;11:875–81.
7. Wolf EM, Wilk RM, Richmond JC. Arthroscopic Bankart repair using suture anchors. Op Tech Orthop. 1991;1:184–91.
8. Armangil M, Basat HÇ, Akan B, Karaduman M, Demirtas M. Arthroscopic stabilization of anterior shoulder instability using a single anterior portal. Acta Orthop Traumatol Turc. 2015;49:6–12.
9. Burks RT, Presson AP, Weng HY. An analysis of technical aspects of the arthroscopic Bankart procedure as performed in the United States. Arthroscopy. 2014;30:1246–53.
10. Elena N, Woodall BM, Ahn S, et al. Anterior shoulder stabilization using a single portal technique with suture lasso. Arthrosc Tech. 2018;7:e505–9.
11. Lavender C, Lycans D, Kopiec A, Sayan A. Nanoscopic single-incision anterior labrum repair. Arthrosc Tech. 2020;9:e297–301.

Single-Incision Rotator Cuff Repair

Galen Berdis and Chad Lavender

1 Introduction

Rotator cuff tears have a high prevalence in the adult population, with increasing incidence with patient age [1]. Initially, open and mini-open repair techniques were developed using bone tunnels, but as technology has advanced, arthroscopic techniques have been developed. Over time, these techniques have been improved on with advances in knot-tying technique, new anchors, suture development, and visualization. Arthroscopic techniques have shown a clear advantage in terms of better patient outcome scores as well as lower complication rates when compared with mini-open techniques [1–4]. Traditionally, an arthroscopic rotator cuff repair is performed with the camera through a viewing portal in the back of the shoulder with as many as three working portals in the lateral and anterior aspect of the shoulder. This chapter describes a single-incision rotator cuff repair technique using the NanoScope (Arthrex, Naples, FL) to eliminate the posterior viewing portal as well as all but one of the working portals to complete a repair of a full thickness rotator cuff tear. We feel there are distinct advantages to this technique, including decreased fluid necessary for the repair, which would decrease postoperative pain, and potentially leading to improved outcomes after surgery.

With Permission from Arthroscopy Techniques Lavender, Chad et al. "Single-Incision Rotator Cuff Repair With a Needle Arthroscope." *Arthroscopy techniques* vol. 9,4 e419-e423. 3 Mar. 2020, doi:https://doi.org/10.1016/j.eats.2019.11.012

G. Berdis
PGY4 Marshall University, Scott Depot, WV, USA

C. Lavender (✉)
Orthopaedic Surgery Sports Medicine, Marshall University, Scott Depot, WV, USA

C. Lavender (ed.), *Biologic and Nanoarthroscopic Approaches in Sports Medicine*, https://doi.org/10.1007/978-3-030-71323-2_15

2 Indications

This technique is most useful for small full thickness tears which are treated with a single row type repair in our practice.

3 Contraindications

In larger tears where a complete double row repair is necessary, the NanoScope could still be used but further working portals would need to be established. Larger tears may require more flow, but the NanoScope could still be utilized in the repair.

4 Surgical Technique

4.1 Patient Setup

The patient is placed in the lateral decubitus position with the operative extremity placed in a standard lateral arm positioner. An axillary roll is placed under the non-operative extremity, and all bony prominences are well padded. The operative shoulder landmarks are marked out including the scapular spine, acromion, coracoid, clavicle, and acromioclavicular joint.

4.2 Needle Arthroscope Insertion

A spinal needle with trocar is inserted into the glenohumeral joint posteriorly (Fig. 15.1). The trocar is removed from the spinal needle, and a nitinol wire is inserted into the needle. The needle is removed with retention of nitinol wire within

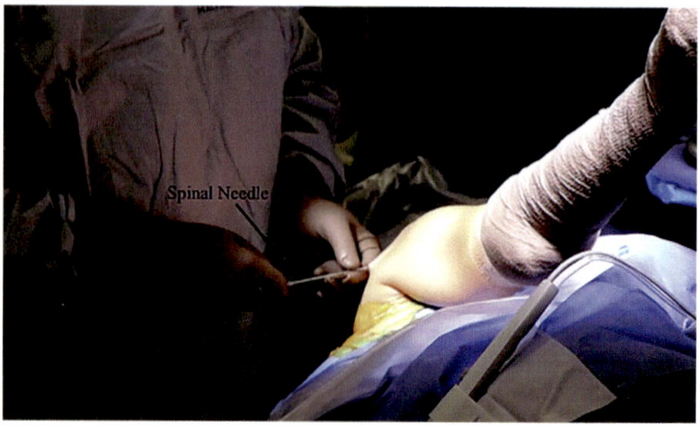

Fig. 15.1 Viewing the right shoulder from outside of the joint with a spinal needle inserted posteriorly

the needle tract. A 2.7-mm cannula is then inserted over the wire, and the wire is removed. Inflow is then placed onto the cannula and the needle arthroscope is inserted for visualization of the joint (Fig. 15.2). A standard diagnostic arthroscopy is then performed identifying the small full-thickness rotator cuff tear. The tear is then marked with a spinal needle so that it can be easily identified in the subacromial space (Fig. 15.3).

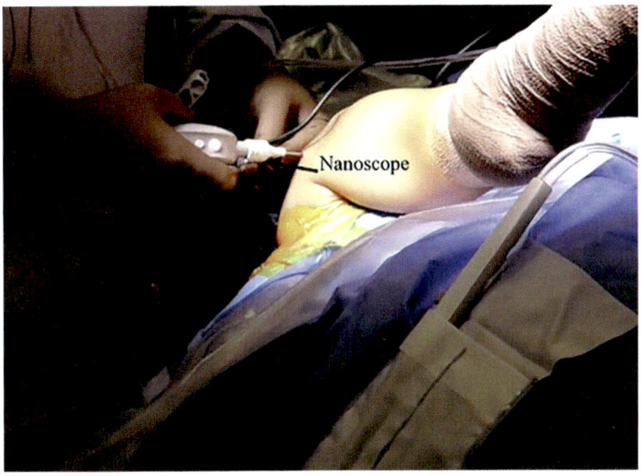

Fig. 15.2 Viewing the right shoulder from outside of the joint, a 2.7-mm cannula is inserted posteriorly and the NanoScope has been placed into the joint

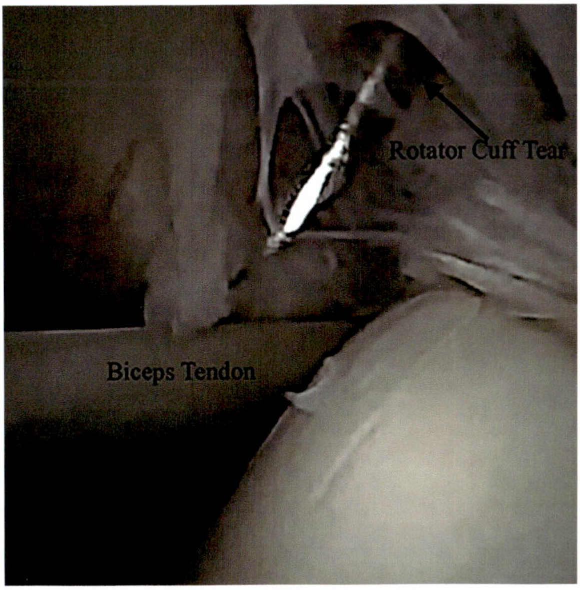

Fig. 15.3 Viewing the right shoulder glenohumeral joint posteriorly with the 0° NanoScope, the rotator cuff tear is seen and marked with a spinal needle

4.3 Lateral Subacromial Portal

The camera is withdrawn and the trocar is inserted into the spinal needle, which is then inserted into the subacromial space via a posterior approach. The trocar is removed, and a nitinol wire is again inserted through the needle. The cannula is inserted over the nitinol wire, and the camera is inserted into the cannula. A spinal needle is used from a lateral approach to localize the lateral working portal. A small incision is then made and a standard 6-mm cannula (Arthrex) is inserted for working purposes. The inflow is then switched to this lateral portal to allow better inflow.

4.4 Rotator Cuff Repair

A 4.5-mm shaver (Arthrex) is then used through the lateral portal to perform a minimal bursectomy and rotator cuff debridement at the site of the tear (Figs. 15.4 and 15.5). The rotator cuff tear is identified by finding the previously placed spinal needle. Once adequate visualization has been achieved with the shaver, a looped FiberLink suture (Arthrex) is then placed into the rotator cuff tear using a scorpion device (Arthrex) through the lateral portal (Fig. 15.6). Next, suture tape (Arthrex) is placed into the anterior limb of the rotator cuff tear (Fig. 15.7). The inferior limb is then retrieved through the lateral portal, and using the scorpion (Arthrex), it is placed through the posterior portion of the tear. This gives an inverted mattress stitch. All three suture tails are brought out laterally and placed into a 4.75 swivel

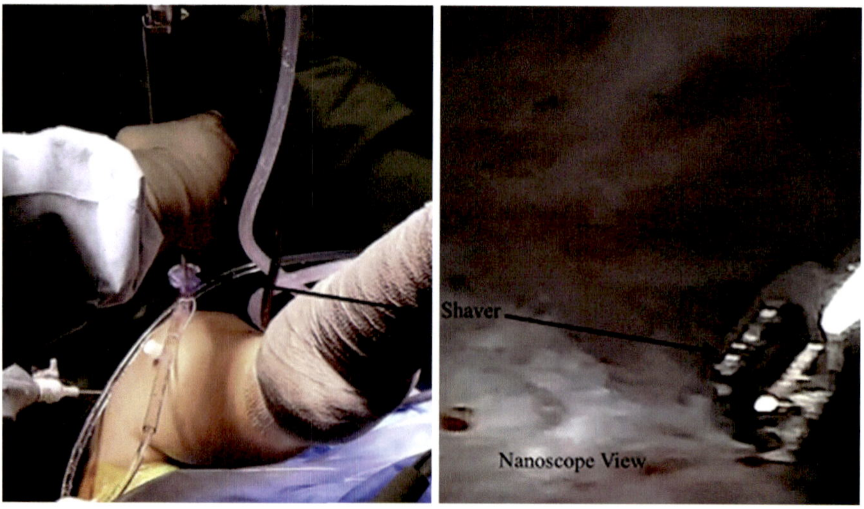

Fig. 15.4 Viewing the right shoulder with two separate views. The view on the left is from outside of the joint showing the NanoScope posteriorly and the shaver coming in laterally. The view on the right is viewing from posteriorly with the Nanoscope and the shaver is seen coming in from laterally

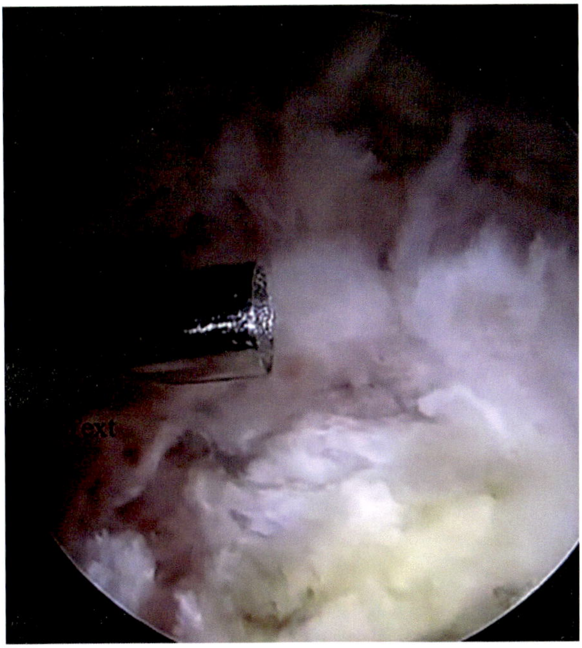

Fig. 15.5 Viewing the right shoulder laterally with the 30° arthroscope, the NanoScope can be seen coming in from posteriorly

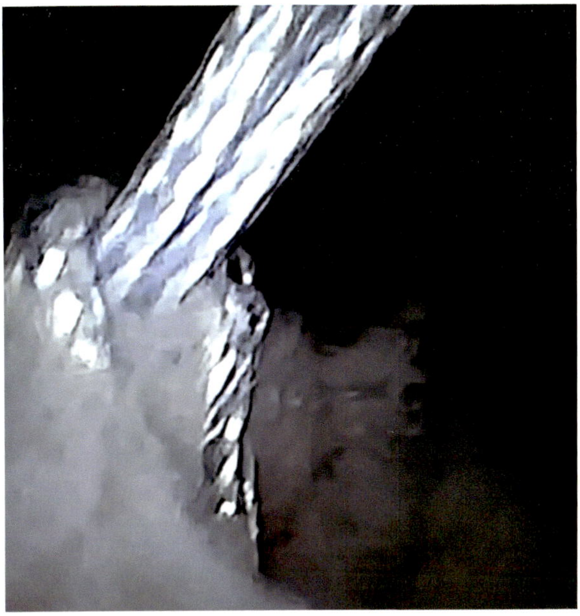

Fig. 15.6 Viewing the right shoulder subacromial joint posteriorly with the 0° NanoScope, the FiberLink (Arthrex) can be seen placed into the rotator cuff tear

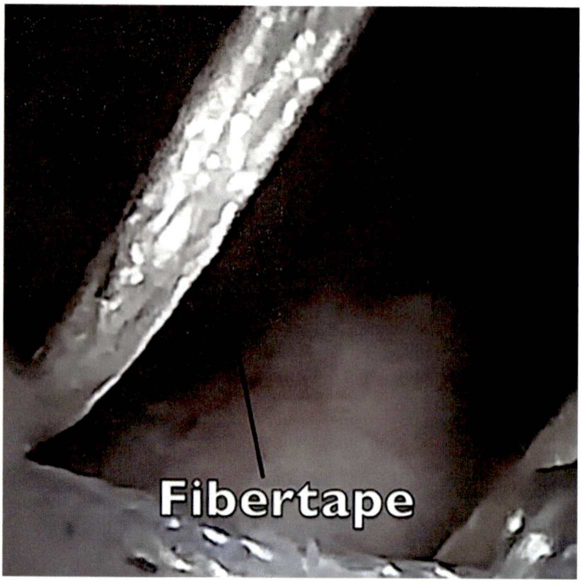

Fig. 15.7 Viewing the right shoulder subacromial joint posteriorly using the 0° NanoScope, the FiberTape suture (Arthrex) can be seen placed into the rotator cuff

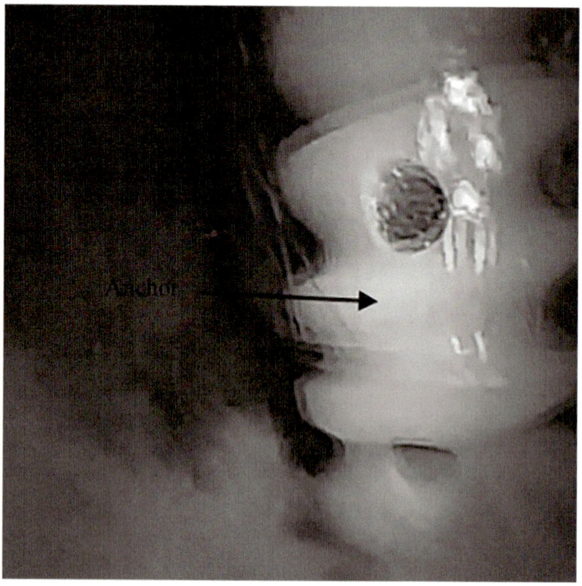

Fig. 15.8 Viewing the right shoulder subacromial joint posteriorly using the 0° NanoScope, the 4.75 swivel lock anchor (Arthrex) can be seen being inserted into the humerus

lock anchor (Arthrex). A punch is then used to prepare the bone, and the anchor is placed with standard tension (Fig. 15.8). The repair is reviewed from both the posterior portal as well as the lateral portal to ensure adequate repair has been achieved (Fig. 15.9). The instruments are withdrawn, and the portals are closed in a standard fashion (Fig. 15.10).

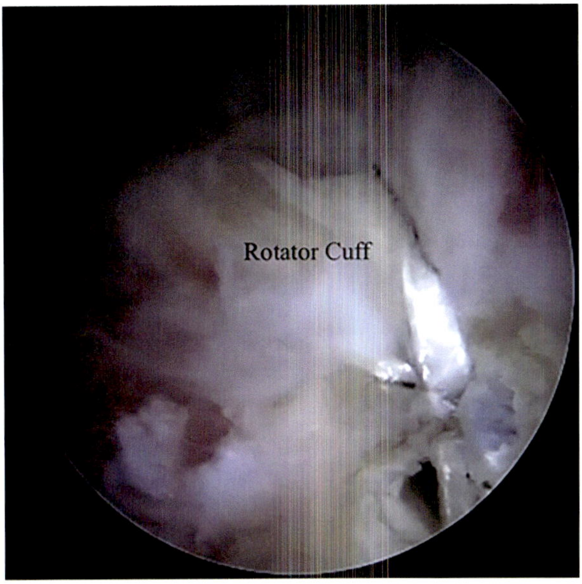

Fig. 15.9 Viewing the right shoulder from laterally using the 30° arthroscope the final rotator cuff repair can be seen

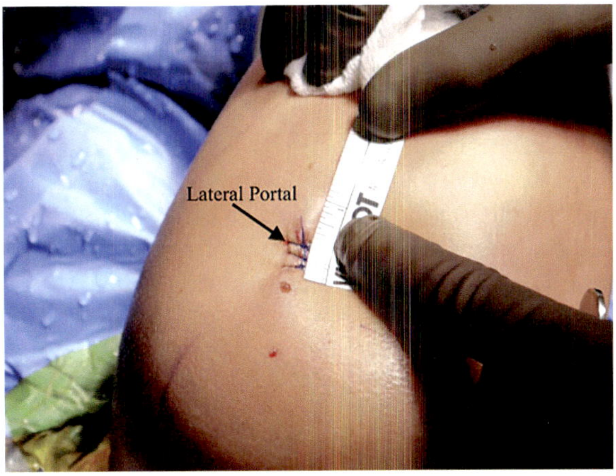

Fig. 15.10 View of the right shoulder from outside the joint in the lateral position seeing there is only a single lateral incision

5 Discussion

Although shoulder arthroscopy has led to improvements in patient-related outcomes in rotator cuff repair, many patients continue having shoulder pain and swelling for some time after arthroscopy. Multiple portals into the shoulder allow for fluid extravasation, causing significant swelling in the shoulder, which irritates soft tissues. In addition, repeated insertion of instruments through the muscle and fascia can cause trauma to the area, leading to more pain postoperatively. The technique described here uses needle arthroscopy to minimize the trauma to the posterior joint capsule and infraspinatus for initial diagnostic arthroscopy. A minimal bursectomy in the subacromial space allows for the retention of a major blood and stem cell supply to the rotator cuff [5]. A single lateral incision is then used with a cannula to minimize damage to the lateral shoulder, and when properly placed, allows for a complete repair of the damaged tendon to the bone [6].

Patient selection is critical when attempting to use this technique, as indications are limited. Current indications are listed in Table 1. This technique is difficult until the surgeon is comfortable using the instruments and the 0-degree scope. Pearls and pitfalls associated with the technique are described in Table 2. The technique is limited by the size, shape, and location of the tear. The small cannula limits the amount of fluid inflow into the shoulder, which can be an advantage due to less swelling and potentially less pain immediately postoperatively. Less inflow also decreases visualization due to less pressure in the shoulder and subacromial space during the procedure. This can lead to an increased propensity for bleeding during the procedure. Performing a small bursectomy has shown to help with the propensity for bleeding, and allows for minimal trauma to the tissue. A larger or retracted tear would be very difficult to repair using the technique described above as more exposure is needed. The 0-degree design of the arthroscope provides a 120-degree field of view but does limit the surgeon's ability to change viewing angles without changing the viewing site. Adding portal sites can improve the access into the subacromial space for larger tears, and with more experience using these instruments, repair of a larger tear would be feasible. Isolated repair of a rotator cuff tear is possible using the technique described above, but if other procedures were needed during arthroscopy such as a subscapularis repair, arthroscopic biceps tenodesis, or distal clavicle excision for acromioclavicular arthritis, a standard arthroscope would most likely be required. Increased surgeon experience with the technique and experience will also yield improved efficiency with the procedure as well as increased indications for the technique. Advantages and disadvantages of using this technique are outlined in Table 3. These include minimal damage to the surrounding tissue.

Table 1 Current indications and relative contraindications for needle arthroscopy of the shoulder

Indications
Partial thickness, isolated bursal sided or articular sided rotator cuff tears
Small, non-retracted isolated full thickness rotator cuff tears
Relative contraindications
Larger or retracted rotator cuff tears
Rotator cuff or labral surgery requiring concomitant procedures such as arthroscopic biceps tenodesis, distal clavicle excision, subscapularis repair

Table 2 Pearls and pitfalls of the single-incision rotator cuff repair

Pearls
Inflow should be switched to the lateral portal to allow more flow
Limited bursectomy creates decreased bleeding which improves visualization
The 30° arthroscope can be switched to the lateral portal to get a direct view of the tear.
Pitfalls
Improper placement of the posterior spinal needle can cause difficult visualization

Table 3 Advantages and disadvantages of the single-incision rotator cuff repair

Advantages	
	Decreased loss and need for fluid less swelling and pain
	Possible increase in early motion
Disadvantages	
	Additional cost of NanoScope
	Difficult viewing angles
	Decreased and/or difficult visualization

There is less inflow of arthroscopic fluid, leading to less swelling and potentially less pain in the immediate postoperative period. This, in turn, should allow for easier and faster gains in range of motion. Visualization and arthroscope placement can be technically demanding, but when placed properly, adequate visualization can be achieved. Although this technique can be difficult and has limitations, we feel it has a role in the future of arthroscopy and as we gain experience with needle arthroscopy the indications for its use will increase.

6 Editor's View

As we look at these nanoscopic techniques I think this technique, in particular, is one of the largest repairs that has been done using the NanoScope. It is a single-incision rotator cuff repair based on the percutaneous viewing portal posteriorly. Obviously, less incisions should lead to improved outcomes. It should be noted that you really need to familiarize yourself with the NanoScope before attempting the NanoScope rotator cuff repair as it can be challenging based on your viewing angles. Now that we have the high flow sheath the flow should be improved and less of an issue. I think with larger cuff tears this is also an option because your visualization actually would be easier than in a small tear. In my opinion, the takeaway point is to consider nanoscopic and the most minimally invasive techniques that you can to improve patient outcomes and I look forward to seeing results in the future comparing the nanoscopic rotator cuff repair versus standard arthroscopic rotator cuff repairs.

References

1. Tashjian RZ. Epidemiology, natural history, and indications for treatment of rotator cuff tears. Clin. Sports Med. 2012;31:589–604.
2. Liu J, Fan L, Zhu Y, Yu H, Xu T, Li G. Comparison of clinical outcomes in all-arthroscopic versus mini-open repair of rotator cuff tears: a randomized clinical trial. Medicine (Baltimore). 2017;96:e6322.
3. Osti L, Papalia R, Paganelli M, Denaro E, Maffulli N. Arthroscopic vs mini-open rotator cuff repair. A quality of life impairment study. Int. Orthop. 2010;34:389–94.
4. Day M, Westermann R, Duchman K, et al. Comparison of short-term complications after rotator cuff repair: open versus arthroscopic. Arthroscopy. 2018;34:1130–6.
5. Freislederer F, Dittrich M, Scheibel M. Biological augmentation with subacromial bursa in arthroscopic rotator cuff repair. Arthrosc. Tech. 2019;8:e741–7.
6. Lavender C, et al. Single-incision rotator cuff repair with a needle arthroscope. Arthrosc Tech. 2020;9(4):e419–23. https://doi.org/10.1016/j.eats.2019.11.012.

Incisionless Synovectomy of the Knee

Tyag K. Patel and John Jasko

1 Introduction

Synovectomy of the knee is a procedure that has multiple indications of which the most common are septic arthritis, inflammatory arthritis, and synovial tumors. The procedure is done through either an open or an arthroscopic approach; however, an incisionless method using a Nanoscope (Arthrex, Naples, FL) can also be utilized. With the incisionless method, a Graftnet (Arthrex, Naples, FL) allows tissue from the synovium to be collected and evaluated which can aid in diagnosis and treatment. Septic arthritis of the knee is a surgical emergency and is one of the more common reasons to perform a synovectomy. Once septic arthritis is diagnosed, urgent surgical debridement along with antibiotic treatment is critical. Surgical decompression reduces the intra-articular burden of bacteria and removes harmful debris released from the host inflammatory response. Panjawani et al. conducted a systematic review and meta-analysis to compare reoperation rates, length of stay, and functional outcome between arthroscopy and open arthrotomy of septic native knees [1]. They found seven studies of which 723 patients underwent arthroscopic I&D and 366 patients underwent open I&D. The relative risk of reoperation and LOS of stay was lower in the arthroscopy group, and one study reported better functional outcomes with arthroscopy. The authors concluded arthroscopic debridement results in lower risk of re-operation than open arthrotomy. Furthermore, in a retrospective study of one institution, Johns et al. compared open to arthroscopic

With permission from Arthroscopy Techniques: Lavender C, Patel T, Adil Syed, Blickenstaff B, Oliashirazi A. Incisionless Knee Synovectomy and Biopsy With Needle Arthroscope and Autologous Tissue Collector. *Arthroscopy Techniques*, Vol 9, No 9 (September), 2020; pp. e1259–1262.

T. K. Patel (✉)
Marshall University, Orthopedic Surgery, Huntington, WV, USA

J. Jasko
Marshall University, Orthopaedic Surgery Sports Medicine, Huntington, WV, USA

C. Lavender (ed.), *Biologic and Nanoarthroscopic Approaches in Sports Medicine*, https://doi.org/10.1007/978-3-030-71323-2_16

I&D of native knees [2]. They included 166 knees of which 123 knees were treated with arthroscopic I&D while 43 knees were treated with open I&D. They found 71% of open I&D and 50% of arthroscopic I&D required repeat irrigation. In addition, the arthroscopic groups had a lower total number of irrigation procedures, better mean post op ROM ($p < 0.05$). In regards to PVNS, arthroscopy has also been found to have similar recurrence and complication rates to open approaches [3, 4]. The following technique describes an incisionless approach for synovectomy and biopsy of the knee that can be used for the diagnosis and/or treatment of septic arthritis, inflammatory arthritis, and synovial tumors.

2 Indications

Patients with suspected septic knee, synovial tumors, or disease processes in which you would like a biopsy and synovectomy. Compromised patients at high risk and those in the intensive care setting.

3 Contraindications

Patients which require larger resections and those which have failed previous synovectomys.

4 Surgical Technique

4.1 Patient Setup

The patient is placed in the supine position with the operative extremity in a leg holder and a tourniquet applied to the operative thigh. The non-operative extremity is placed over a well-padded pillow in slight flexion. The operative extremity is exsanguinated, and the tourniquet is inflated.

4.2 Nanoscope Insertion

A spinal needle is inserted into anterolateral joint space while the knee is in full extension. The knee may need slight flexion to allow entry into the patellofemoral joint. A nitinol wire is inserted into the needle and the needle is removed. A small 2.7 mm cannula is then inserted over the wire and the wire is removed (Fig. 1). Care should be taken when inserting the 2.7 cannula as it can cause cartilage damage during insertion (Fig. 2). Inflow is then placed onto the cannula and the Nanoscope (Arthrex, Naples, FL) is inserted for visualization of the joint. A standard diagnostic arthroscopy is then performed in the patellofemoral joint. The Nanoscope is then redirected into the medial joint space. Rather than gliding into the medial joint as is

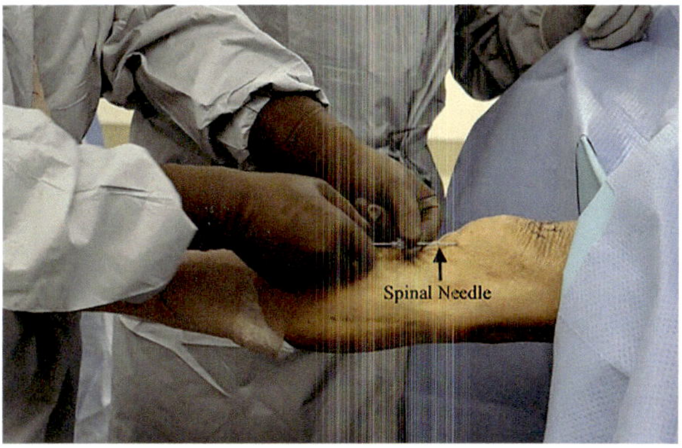

Fig. 1 View of a left knee from outside the knee. The spinal needle is seen inserted into the patellofemoral joint while the knee is in full extension

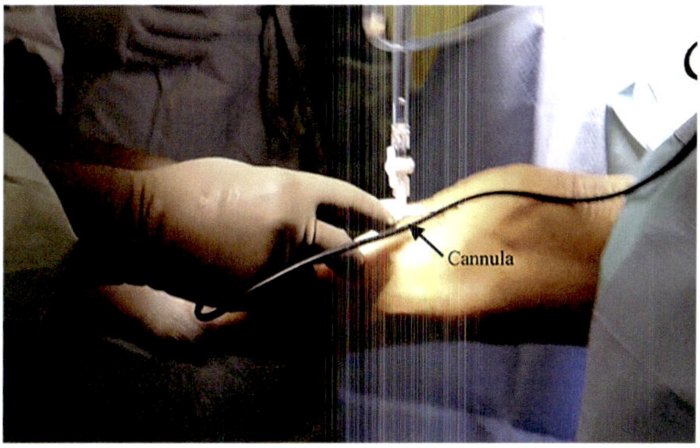

Fig. 2 View of a left knee in the extended position from outside the knee. The cannula has been inserted into the knee with the Nanoscope inserted

done with standard arthroscopy, it can be helpful to come out slightly and redirect into the space.

4.3 Medial Portal

An 18-gauge spinal needle is then used to localize the medial portal location in an outside fashion. A nitinol wire is inserted into the needle and the needle is removed (Fig. 3). A small 2.7 mm cannula is then inserted over the wire and the wire is removed.

4.4 Synovectomy

The Nanoscope is then redirected into the patellofemoral joint and a NanoShaver (Arthrex, Naples, FL) is used to perform the synovectomy through the medial portal. Alternatively, a 3 mm shaver can be used for a more aggressive option (Fig. 4). The Graftnet is then applied to the shaver to collect tissue for analysis (Figs. 5 and 6). The shaver is then brought to the medial compartment to then be

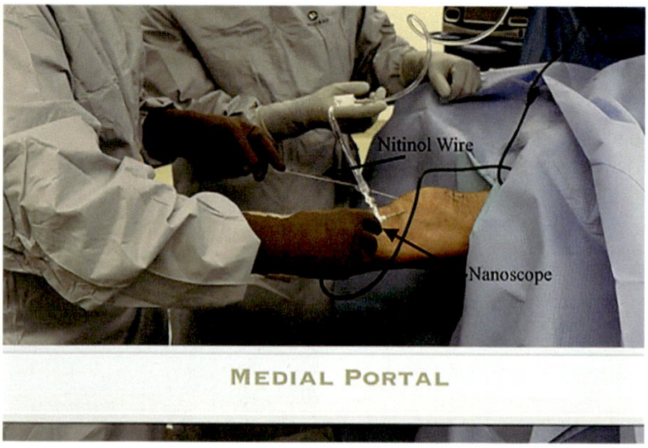

Fig. 3 View of a left knee from outside the knee with the knee in full extension. The medial portal has been established with a nitinol wire inserted into a spinal needle while the Nanoscope is in the anterolateral portal and the knee is in full extension

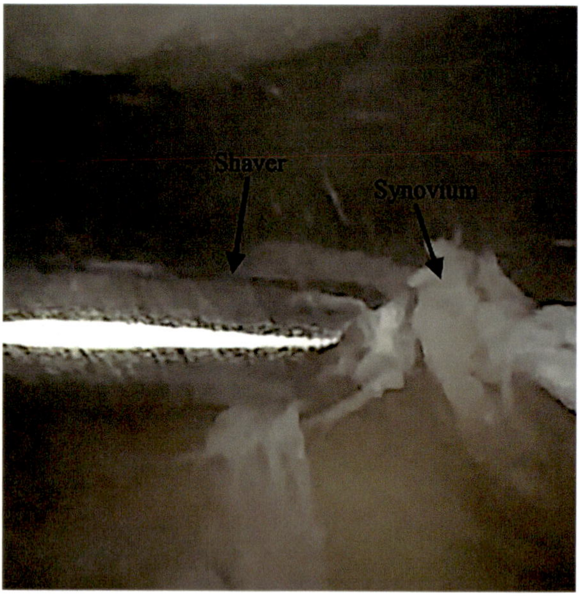

Fig. 4 View of a left knee in the extended position with the 0 degrees Nanoscope from the anterolateral portal. The shaver has been placed in the medial portal with the knee in full extension. The shaver is harvesting synovial tissue

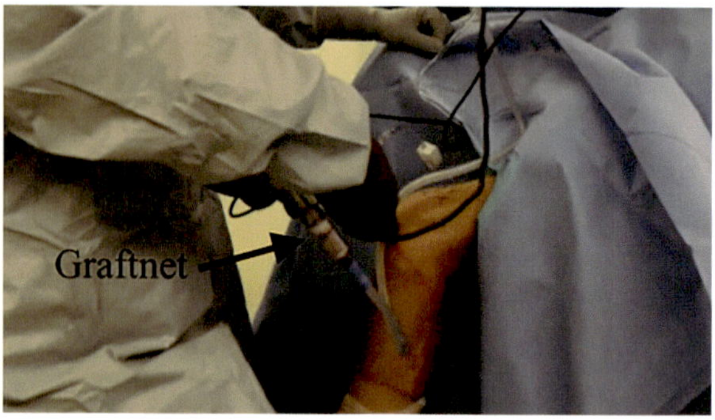

Fig. 5 View of a left knee in 90 degrees of flexion. The Graftnet has been attached to the shaver while the shaver is in the anterolateral portal

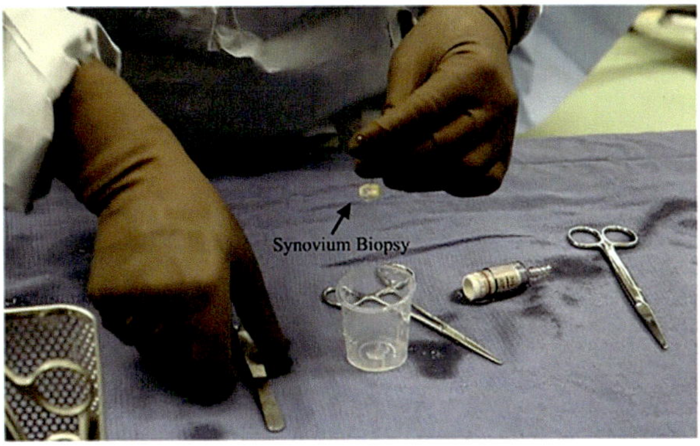

Fig. 6 The synovial tissue has been removed from the Graftnet and is being placed into a sterile cup and submitted for pathologic evaluation

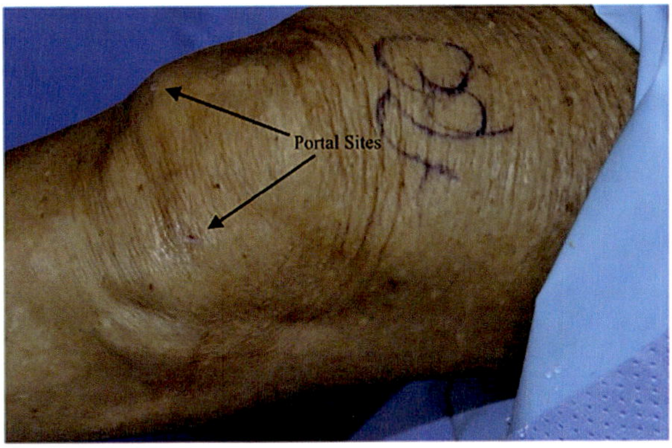

Fig. 7 View of a left knee in full extension. The portal sites are seen on the front of the knee

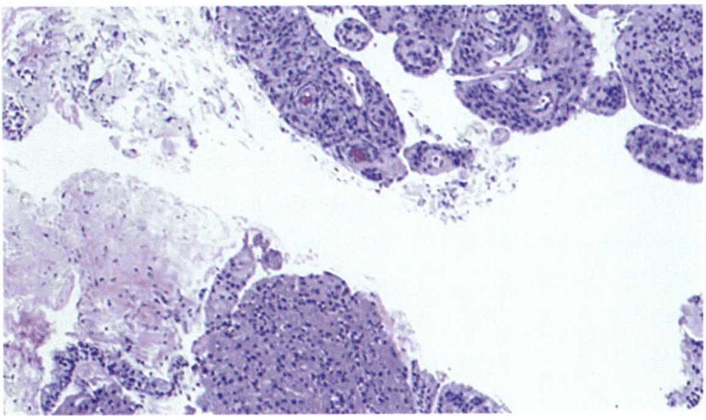

Fig. 8 Final pathologic findings showing the synovium and the maintained cellular architecture after biopsy using the Graftnet. Hematoxylin and eosin stain with original magnification ×200

used to debride the medial compartment. Next, the Nanoscope is switched to the medial compartment and the shaver can be brought in laterally to complete the synovectomy anteriorly, laterally, and in the patellofemoral joint. Finally, tissue obtained from the Graftnet is then placed into a sterile cup and sent to pathology for evaluation (Figs. 7 and 8).

5 Discussion

Synovectomy can be done through an open incision or arthroscopically, and here we describe an incisionless arthroscopic technique using the Nanoscope. The Nanoscope needle arthroscopy system is both diagnostic and therapeutic. It allows direct visualization of intra-articular pathology and its use in combination with the Graftnet allows for recovery of tissue for histologic analysis. In addition, it eliminates the need for incisions, requiring only a spinal needle to establish access to the joint. The most common indications for synovectomy include septic arthritis, inflammatory arthritis, and synovial tumors. Traditional arthroscopy of knees offers several advantages including magnified view, better access to harder to reach areas of the knee and more visibility of gutters, as well as the high flow of normal saline in a closed cavity allowing for dislodgement of any necrotic material or pus [5]. There are limitations to the nanoscopic technique similar to those previously described for other nanoscopic techniques which include technical difficulty using the 0-degree lens, difficult visualization due to flow, and the need for the more precise location of portal sites [6]. Pearls of this technique include redirecting the Nanoscope when entering into different compartments, and using a 3 mm shaver for improved suction and debridement [7]. Risks of this technique include articular cartilage damage from the sharper trochar and missing joint pathology because of the decreased visualization due to flow and smaller size of the arthroscope. Finally, minimally invasive surgery results in reduced pain, swelling, complications, and a quicker recovery – therefore this technique should improve patient results and should especially be considered when the diagnosis is questioned or in critically ill patients where an incisionless approach is favored.

6 Editors View

This chapter describes another one of our incisionless techniques. This technique in particular is useful especially in a sick or compromised patient with a possible or probable knee infection to treat the infection in as minimally invasive fashion as possible. Also, it is very useful for diagnostic purposes that can easily be used in a setting of tumor pathology or other undiagnosed problems within the knee. I personally use the Nanoscope in many diagnostic cases at this point and feel that it is a very useful tool when combined with the Graftnet incisionless approach to correctly diagnose intra-articular pathologies of the knee. It is very exciting to see where we are with nano arthroscopy and combining that with some of the minimally invasive tools that we have to produce techniques such as this and improve patient outcomes.

References

1. Panjwani T, Wong KL, Tan SHS, Liau G, Vaidya N, Krishna L. Arthroscopic debridement has lower re-operation rates than arthrotomy in the treatment of acute septic arthritis of the knee: a meta-analysis. Journal of ISAKOS: Joint Disorders & Orthopaedic Sports Medicine 2019;(4):307–12.
2. Johns BP, Loewenthal MR, Dewar DC. Open compared with arthroscopic treatment of acute septic arthritis of the native knee. J Bone Joint Surg Am. 2017;99(6):499–505. https://doi.org/10.2106/JBJS.16.00110.
3. Rodriguez-Merchan EC. Review Article: Open versus arthroscopic synovectomy for pigmented villonodular synovitis of the knee. J Orthop Surg. 2014;22(3):406–8.
4. Pan X, Zhang X, Liu Z, Wen H, Mao X. Treatment for chronic synovitis of knee: arthroscopic or open synovectomy. Rheumatol Int. 2012;32:1733–6. https://doi.org/10.1007/s00296-011-1901-3.
5. Lui TH. Complete arthroscopic synovectomy in management of recalcitrant septic arthritis of the knee joint. Arthrosc Tech. 2017;6(2):e467–e475 137.
6. Lavender C, et al. Nanoscopic single-incision anterior labrum repair. Arthrosc Tech. 2020;9:e297.
7. Lavender C, Patel T, Syed A, Blickenstaff B, Oliashirazi A. Incisionless knee synovectomy and biopsy with needle arthroscope and autologous tissue collector. Arthrosc Tech. 2020;9(9):e1259–62.

Incisionless Synovium and Bone Biopsy of a Painful Total Knee Arthroplasty

Syed Ali Sina Adil, Matthew Bullock, and Ali Oliashirazi

1 Introduction

Synovium and bone biopsy of the knee is a procedure that has been well-described utilizing various arthroscopic and open procedures. Indications for such knee procedures include septic arthritis, inflammatory conditions, and synovial tumors. The diagnosis of periprosthetic joint infection (PJI) is sometimes difficult, occasionally requiring a histological sample when arthrocentesis is inconclusive. Collecting synovial samples has been described by utilizing various arthroscopy portals. Even with the newest arthroscopic approaches obtaining tissue samples has been difficult. For our technique, we combine a more minimally invasive nanoscopic approach with a GraftNet (Arthrex, Naples, FL) to harvest the tissue.

The NanoScope (Arthrex, Naples, FL) is an advanced miniaturized arthroscope with a single-use camera opposite a 1.9-mm diameter viewing cannula that can be inserted into a joint without the need of a traditional incision. In addition to lower blood loss, shorter procedure time, and the potential for quicker recovery, the NanoScope enables a minimally invasive procedure thus decreasing the chance of contamination of a prosthetic joint. The NanoScope has been gaining momentum as an option in the office setting as opposed to the traditional operating room setting thus lowering the associated cost of such a procedure. When combined with the

With permission Lavender et al. Incisionless Synovial and Bone Biopsy of a Painful Total Knee Arthroplasty. *Arthroscopy Techniques*. 2021

S. A. S. Adil
PGY3 Marshall University, Scott Depot, WV, USA

M. Bullock (✉)
Department of Orthopaedic Surgery, Marshall University, Huntington, WV, USA
e-mail: bullockm@marshall.edu

A. Oliashirazi
Marshall University, Scott Depot, WV, USA

C. Lavender (ed.), *Biologic and Nanoarthroscopic Approaches in Sports Medicine*, https://doi.org/10.1007/978-3-030-71323-2_17

GraftNet we can obtain significant amounts of tissue without an incision and without damaging or creating contamination to a possibly sterile prosthetic joint.

Most of the literature regarding arthroscopic synovium biopsy and synovectomy has centered around native knee infections. Panjawani et al. [1] conducted a systematic review and meta-analysis to compare outcomes between arthroscopy and arthrotomy of septic native knees [1]. Seven studies included 723 patients underwent arthroscopic irrigation and debridement (I&D) while 366 patients underwent open I&D. The relative risk of reoperation was significantly lower in the arthroscopy group, while the length of stay was lower in the arthroscopy group in all included studies, and one study reported better functional outcomes with arthroscopy. Peres et al. [2] performed a randomized control trial comparing arthrotomy versus arthroscopy in the treatment of knee septic arthritis. They concluded both techniques had similar effectiveness in healing with arthroscopy yielding lower infection rate and lower inflammatory reaction. Furthermore, in a retrospective study of one institution, Johns et al. [3] compared open to arthroscopic I&D of native knees. They included 166 knees with 123 treated with arthroscopic I&D and 43 treated with open I&D. They found 71% of open I&D and 50% of arthroscopic I&D required repeat irrigation. In addition, the arthroscopic groups had a lower total number of irrigation procedures, better mean postop range-of-motion ($p < 0.05$).

2 Indications

Patients with a total knee arthroplasty which is "possibly infected" such as those with an MSIS score of 2–5.

3 Contraindications

Patients with an obvious prosthetic joint infection which should be treated open and those which are obviously not infected and have been completely negative on work up.

4 Surgical Technique

4.1 Patient Setup

The patient is placed in the supine position with the left (operative) extremity in a leg holder and a tourniquet applied to the operative thigh. The non-operative extremity is placed over a well-padded pillow in slight flexion. The operative extremity is exsanguinated and the tourniquet is inflated.

4.2 Nanoscope Insertion

A spinal needle is inserted into superolateral joint space while the knee is in full extension. A nitinol wire is inserted into the needle and the needle is removed (Fig. 1). A high flow 3.4 mm cannula is then inserted over the wire and the wire is removed. Care should be taken when inserting the 3.4 cannula as it can cause damage during insertion. Inflow is then placed onto the cannula and the NanoScope (Arthrex) is inserted for visualization of the joint. A standard diagnostic arthroscopy is then performed in the patellofemoral joint. Alternatively, you could begin by placing the NanoScope portal in the anterolateral portal; however, we recommend establishing this portal which can be used later as a working portal. The other portals will be in the anterolateral joint space and anteromedial joint space and will be established in a similar fashion with the knee in flexion (Fig. 2).

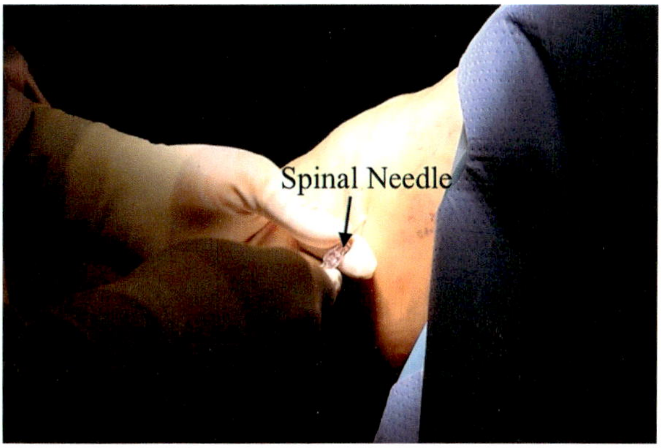

Fig. 1 With the knee in the extension you can see a spinal needle with a nitinol wire being placed through the needle into the superolateral aspect of the patellofemoral joint

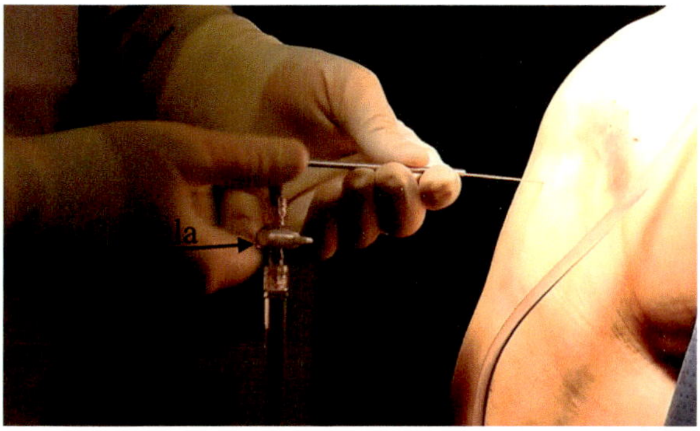

Fig. 2 With the knee in flexion a high flow cannula can be seen placed into the anterolateral portal

4.3 Diagnostic Arthroscopy

Using the NanoScope through the superolateral portal and the knee in extension the patellofemoral synovium is examined and found to be hypertrophic, hypervascularized, and inflamed. The NanoScope is then placed through the anterolateral joint space through the high flow cannula and the patellofemoral joint is viewed and examined.

4.4 Synovium Biopsy

Viewing through the anterolateral joint space with the knee in extension a shaver is placed through the superolateral joint space. The GraftNet is attached to the shaver and synovium biopsies are obtained. Care is taken to obtain samples from the medial aspect, lateral aspect, and superior aspect (Fig. 3). Next, a shaver with the GraftNet is placed through the anteromedial portal and further biopsies can be obtained. The knee is then brought to flexion and after using the anteromedial portal as the working portal the shaver is placed through the anterolateral portal and the anterior synovium is biopsied. Care is taken to view the tibial–cement interface and anterior compartment.

4.5 Bone Biopsy

Placing the NanoScope through the anterolateral portal and shaver through the superior lateral portal areas on the lateral bone interface and anterior flange bone interface are shaved down to bone. Then the GraftNet is applied to the shaver and bone biopsies are obtained. First, we take the biopsy from the lateral femur then the anterior bone is biopsied (Figs. 4, 5, 6, and 7). Care must be made not to resect too much bone.

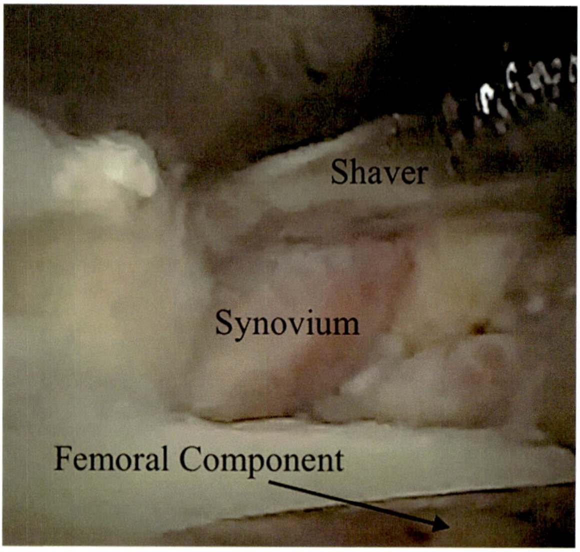

Fig. 3 With the patient supine and the knee in extension we are viewing with a 0° Nanoscope from the anterolateral portal and the shaver is seen coming in percutaneously through the superior lateral portal performing the patellofemoral synovium biopsy

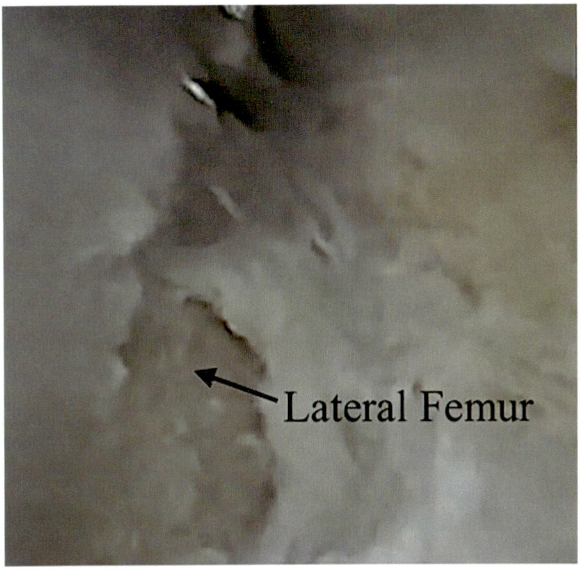

Fig. 4 With the patient supine and the knee in extension we are viewing with a 0° Nanoscope from the anterolateral portal and the shaver is seen coming in percutaneously through the superior lateral portal performing the lateral bone biopsy

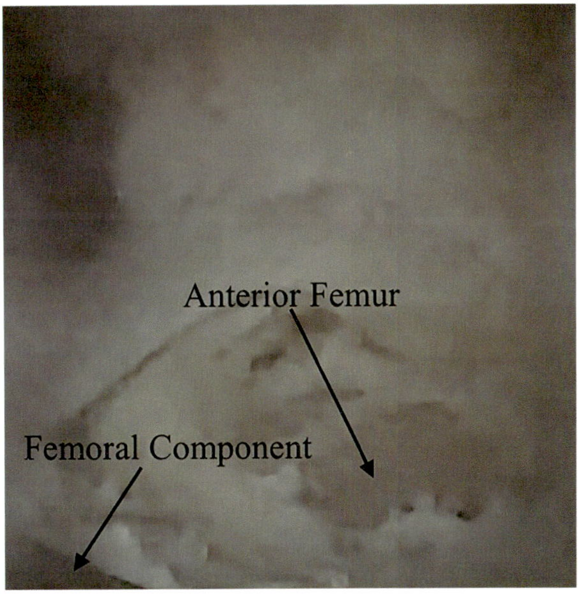

Fig. 5 With the patient supine and the knee in extension we are viewing with a 0° Nanoscope from the anterolateral portal and the anterior femur is seen after the bone biopsy has been performed

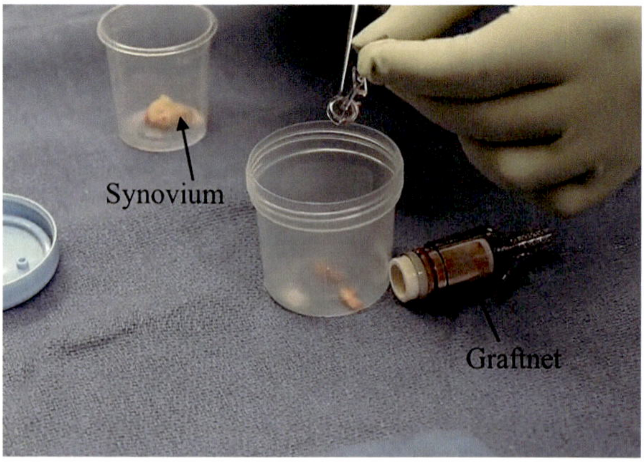

Fig. 6 The GraftNet is seen on the table and synovium biopsies are placed into sterile cups

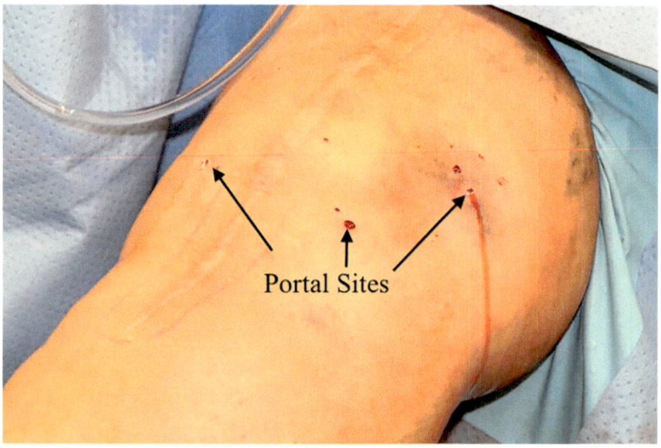

Fig. 7 The patient is supine and the knee is seen in full extension with only small portal sites and no incisions

5 Discussion

The criteria for the diagnosis of periprosthetic joint infection (PJI) after total knee arthroplasty have been established and updated in 2018 by the Musculoskeletal Infection Society (MSIS). The criteria are as follows: two positive cultures or the presence of a sinus tract are considered as major criteria and diagnostic of PJI. The calculated weights of an elevated serum CRP (>1 mg/dL), D-dimer (>860 ng/mL), and erythrocyte sedimentation rate (>30 mm/h) are 2, 2, and 1 points, respectively. Furthermore, elevated synovial fluid white blood cell count (>3000 cells/μL), alpha-defensin (signal-to-cutoff ratio > 1), leukocyte esterase (++), polymorphonuclear percentage (>80%), and synovial CRP (>6.9 mg/L) are 3, 3, 3, 2, and 1 points, respectively. Patients with an aggregate score of greater than or equal to 6 were considered infected, while a score between 2 and 5 required the inclusion of intra-operative findings for confirming or refuting the diagnosis. Intraoperative findings of positive histology, purulence, and single positive culture were assigned 3, 3, and

2 points, respectively. Combined with the preoperative score, a total of greater than or equal to 6 was considered infected, a score between 4 and 5 was inconclusive, and a score of 3 or less was not infected [4–6].

In patients with a score of 2–5 or "possibly infected" according to the MSIS criteria, the use of an updated technique catered to prosthetic joints similar to that previously described in native knees by Lavender et al. is appropriate [7]. In this chapter, we described a novel technique in which a NanoScope and a GraftNet were used to obtain synovium and bone tissue samples in a patient with prior TKA. The goal of the biopsy was to aid in the diagnosis of possible culture-negative infection or inflammatory pathology causing knee pain and swelling. The incidence of culture-negative infection varies from 5 to 42%, and patients are at higher risk for this if given antimicrobial therapy prior to cultures [8]. Obtaining a synovium biopsy through an incisionless technique can be done with low morbidity compared to an open irrigation and debridement to obtain tissue samples. There are several pearls to our technique which make it more simple and effective. It is helpful to use the high-flow nanoscopic cannula for inflow and a larger 3.0 shaver percutaneously to obtain tissue (Table 1). Disadvantages to the technique are that it most likely requires anesthesia and a patient with a likely infection could be treated and diagnosed in one setting versus the diagnostic procedure we describe. Other disadvantages are possible infection if the knee was not infected and this technique can be technically difficult (Table 2). Finally, in patients with significant co-morbidities and at high risk for complications from a large knee procedure, nanoscopic

Table 1 Pearls and pitfalls of the incisionless synovium and biopsy

Pearls
A nanoscopic high-flow cannula should be used to increase flow
Using a 3.0 shaver percutaneously through one of your portals prevents the need for larger incisions
Take at least 3 synovium and 1 bone biopsy
Pitfalls
Take care not to debride too much bone from the anterior bone–cement interface
Using too much suction can decrease visualization

Table 2 Advantages and disadvantages of the incisionless synovium and biopsy

Advantages
Allows tissue diagnosis in a minimally invasive approach
Can be used in sick patients that may be intubated or in the ICU to help with diagnosis
Less contamination of the joint than an open approach
Disadvantages
Most likely requires anesthesia and a trip to the operating room
Possibility of infection in a knee that may not be infected
Technically difficult for surgeons not comfortable with standard arthroscopy

synovectomy, and I&D is an attractive alternative with diagnostic value, lower blood loss, and shorter operating time.

A minimally invasive view from a NanoScope enables the surgeon to inspect the prosthetic knee joint. Important information can be obtained in regard to the polyethylene locking mechanism, bone–cement–implant interface, and prosthetic patellofemoral tracking. Adding the GraftNet to obtain tissue diagnosis may be an increasingly attractive option in those knees which are difficult to diagnose as an infection. We feel this is an advantageous technique in those hard to diagnose painful total knee arthroplasty patients.

6 Editor's View

In my opinion, this technique highlights the versatility of the NanoScope and also the GraftNet which we utilize here for a completely different specialty than sports medicine. This captures the essence of taking minimally invasive surgery and also utilizing the diagnostic capabilities of the GraftNet. This technique could also be utilized in shoulder arthroplasty and you can use the techniques presented here in a variety of cases and patient conditions whenever you need to get a tissue and want to get the tissue in as minimally invasive technique as possible.

References

1. Panjwani T, Wong KL, Tan SHS, et al. Arthroscopic debridement has lower re-operation rates than arthrotomy in the treatment of acute septic arthritis of the knee: a meta-analysis. J ISAKOS: Joint Disord Orthop Sports Med. 2019;4:307–12. https://doi.org/10.1136/jisakos-2018-000269.
2. Peres LR, Marchitto RO, Pereira GS, et al. Arthrotomy versus arthroscopy in the treatment of septic arthritis of the knee in adults: a randomized clinical trial. Knee Surg Sports Traumatol Arthrosc. 2016;24:3155–62. https://doi.org/10.1007/s00167-015-3918-8.
3. Johns BP, Loewenthal MR, Dewar DC. Open compared with arthroscopic treatment of acute septic arthritis of the native knee. J Bone Joint Surg Am. 2017;99:499–505. https://doi.org/10.2106/JBJS.16.00110.
4. Parvizi J, Tan TL, Goswami K, et al. The 2018 definition of periprosthetic hip and knee infection: an evidence-based and validated criteria. J Arthroplast. 2018;33:1309–1314.e2. https://doi.org/10.1016/j.arth.2018.02.078.
5. Van Boxel JA, Paget SA. Predominantly T-cell infiltrate in rheumatoid synovial membranes. N Engl J Med. 1975;293:517–20. https://doi.org/10.1056/NEJM197509112931101.
6. Wasterlain AS, Goswami K, Ghasemi SA, Parvizi J. Diagnosis of periprosthetic infection: recent developments. J Bone Joint Surg Am. 2020;102:1366–75. https://doi.org/10.2106/JBJS.19.00598.
7. Lavender C, Patel T, Adil S, et al. Incisionless knee synovectomy and biopsy with needle arthroscope and autologous tissue collector. Arthrosc Tech. 2020;9:e1259–62. https://doi.org/10.1016/j.eats.2020.05.002.
8. Tande AJ, Patel R. Prosthetic joint infection. Clin Microbiol Rev. 2014;27:302–45. https://doi.org/10.1128/CMR.00111-13.

Nanoscopic Single-Incision Autograft Cartilage Transfer

William Scott Fravel and Baylor Blickenstaff

1 Introduction

Osteochondral defects of the knee (OCD) are due to repetitive microtrauma at the junction of the articular hyaline cartilage and the subchondral bone. Patients may have genetic or other predispositions for the development of these lesions such as vascular injury, trauma, and endocrine disorders [1]. These lesions are most commonly found on the posterolateral aspect of the medial femoral condyle [2]. The prevalence of knee OCD in adults has been estimated to be 15–29 per 100,000 [3, 4]. Diagnosis involves a thorough history detailing onset, history of trauma, past medical history, characterization of pain, and presence of mechanical symptoms. Radiographs will show a lucency on the condyle and MRI can further characterize the stability of the lesion. A period of nonoperative management can be attempted, with anti-inflammatory medicine and nonweight-bearing of the extremity. Failure of nonoperative treatment warrants surgical intervention for improvement in symptoms and prevention of further chondral and subchondral damage to the knee.

Multiple surgical options exist for OCD lesions including debridement with or without microfracture, fixation of the fragment with screws, osteochondral transplant with allograft or autograft, and autologous chondrocyte implantation. The goal of surgical intervention is to fill the defect with cartilage and attempt to recreate a smooth articular surface that can withstand shear and bodyweight forces. Microfracture techniques have been shown to create a more fibrocartilage-type cap over the defect, which is different in biochemical composition than native hyaline

W. S. Fravel · B. Blickenstaff (✉)
Department of Orthopaedic Surgery, Marshall University, Scott Depot, WV, USA
e-mail: blickenstafb@marshall.edu

C. Lavender (ed.), *Biologic and Nanoarthroscopic Approaches in Sports Medicine*, https://doi.org/10.1007/978-3-030-71323-2_18

cartilage. Osteochondral transplant and ACI attempt to fill these defects with hyaline-type cartilage which would allow for a more favorable surface for withstanding the normal forces acting upon the joint. However, there are disadvantages with these two procedures; OATs has the risk of donor site morbidity due to the harvesting of an osteochondral plug, and ACI has historically been an expensive, two-stage surgery requiring harvest of the chondrocytes, shipping to a lab for maturation, and subsequent re-operation for implantation into the defect.

An ideal procedure to treat OCD would allow for hyaline cartilage filling of the lesion with minimal donor-site morbidity and the ability to be performed in a single operation. We have developed a technique that allows for an arthroscopic, single-incision ACT procedure using composite autograft and allograft. Our technique, using the Nanoscope for visualization without an incision for a viewing portal, allows us to prepare the lesion, harvest cartilage autograft, and implant the composite graft in a minimally invasive fashion. This single-stage procedure allows for the filling of the defect without the risks, costs, and hassle of a traditional two-stage ACI procedure. We use the GraftNet to harvest nonarticular cartilage and combine this with autograft BMC and BioCartilage extracellular allograft matrix, creating a composite matrix. The GraftNet is a tissue collector attached to an arthroscopic shaver allowing for simple harvesting of autologous tissue. This composite allows for a hyaline cartilage-like graft to place into the OCD lesion compared to microfracture.

Microfracture surgery has been a useful tool in the treatment of OCD lesions since the 1980s. Steadman et al. reported 80% subjective patient improvement in 1997. Traditional microfracture techniques allow for marrow elements to extrude into the defect, resulting in fibrocartilaginous overgrowth at the lesion site. This fibrocartilage lacks type II collagen as seen in native hyaline cartilage; restoration of more hyaline-like cartilage has been associated with improved clinical outcomes for OCD (DiBartola). BioCartilage is an allograft extracellular matrix containing type II collagen and proteoglycans that is used as a scaffold to augment microfracture. The marrow that is extruded from the microfracture site and interacts with the matrix, allowing for more native-like cartilage formation than microfracture alone. BioCartilage augmentation of OCD lesions has been shown to have better histologic properties after filling than microfracture alone in an animal model (Equine).

Autologous chondrocyte implantation was first reported by Brittberg et al. in 1994. Chondrocytes from non-articulating portions of the knee were harvested, cultured in a lab for up to 3 weeks, and reimplanted via injection into the chondral defect. At 2 years they showed 14 of their 16 patients had good to excellent results. Biopsies were taken of the healed lesions which were of the appearance of hyaline cartilage. The expense of chondrocyte maturation and the nature of needing a second procedure for implantation have given way to research into chondrocyte harvest and implantation as a single procedure. Multiple studies have shown good short-term results with this type of procedure. There are multiple reported techniques, including our own, that show that this may be performed arthroscopically. Recently, we have pushed for our arthroscopy surgeries to become even less invasive by using the Nanoscope for visualization rather than a standard arthroscopic camera. This camera, roughly the size of an 18-gauge needle, can be inserted in multiple areas of the knee to allow visualization without the need for an incision for a standard viewing portal. This chapter describes our single-stage, single-incision ACT procedure of lesion debridement, graft harvest, composite preparation, and graft insertion through a single incision with the Nanoscope for visualization. Used with permission Lavender et al. Nanoscopic Single-Incision Autograft Cartilage Transfer (ACT) Arthroscopy Techniques; Feb 2021 Volume 10 (E545–549).

2 Indications

Full-thickness lesions that extend to subchondral bone are amenable to ACI. Lesions must be contained, found to have a stable rim after debridement, and must have an appropriate height of the cartilage rim allowing containment of the composite graft in the defect. Patients who have failed microfracture, or lesions too large for microfracture.

3 Contraindications

Joint malalignment, multi-compartmental arthritis, and inflammatory arthritis are contraindications to this procedure. Other structural problems such as meniscal or ligamentous pathology that result in increased stress on the lesion site must be addressed at the time of surgery. Smoking and obesity (BMI <35) are contraindications as these factors have been shown to result in worse outcomes with ACI. Age is not a contraindication for ACI; however, some studies have shown that patients <25 years of age have better outcomes than older patients. Patients also must be willing to comply with a strict postoperative rehabilitation regimen [11].

4 Surgical Technique

4.1 Patient Positioning

The patient is placed supine in a standard knee arthroscopy position. The operative extremity is placed into a leg holder with a tourniquet applied to the thigh and the nonoperative extremity is placed on a well-padded leg pillow.

4.2 Bone Marrow Aspiration

Before inflating the tourniquet a small stab incision is made just lateral to the tibial tubercle. An aspiration needle and central sharp trocar are inserted proximally at approximately a 10-degree angle. A mark is made on the needle at 30 mm to avoid over-insertion. Then 60 cc of bone marrow is aspirated into heparinized syringes. This aspiration is concentrated using the Arthrex Angel System to 5 cc of bone marrow concentrate.

4.3 Nanoscope (Arthrex) Insertion

The leg is exsanguinated and a tourniquet is inflated to 250 mm hg. With the operative knee in flexion, a spinal needle is placed in the standard anterolateral portal location. A nitinol wire is inserted through the spinal needle and the needle is removed. Next, the 3.4 mm high-flow Nanoscope cannula (Arthrex) is inserted and the Nanoscope (Arthrex) is inserted into the cannula after the flow is attached. A standard diagnostic arthroscopy is then performed with the Nanoscope.

4.4 Autograft Cartilage Transfer Technique

4.4.1 Lesion Preparation

The lesion on the medial femoral condyle is then identified. A spinal needle is used to establish a standard portal at the location of the medial lesion (Fig. 1). The lesion is prepared and debrided with a shaver and small curette. After the lesion has been prepared a standard microfracture technique is performed with a small drilling device (Powerpick, Arthrex, Inc., Naples, FL) (Fig. 2). First, circumferential perforations are created at the periphery of the lesion, and then central perforations are made down to a bleeding base.

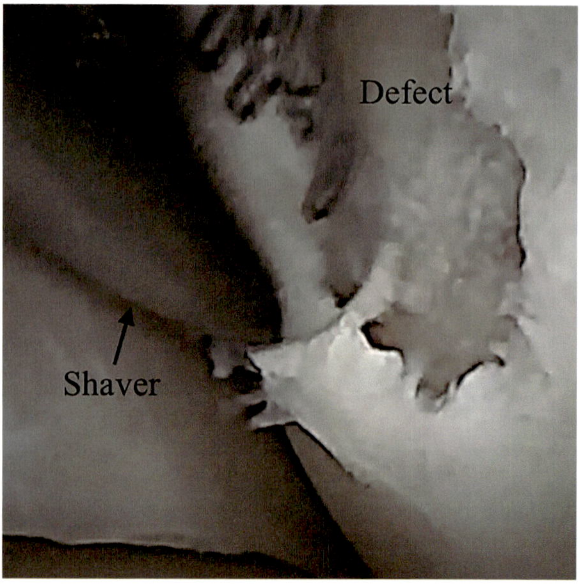

Fig. 1 Viewing the left knee in flexion with the Nanoscope (Arthrex) 0° anterolaterally. The medial femoral defect is seen being prepared by the shaver which is placed through the anteromedial portal

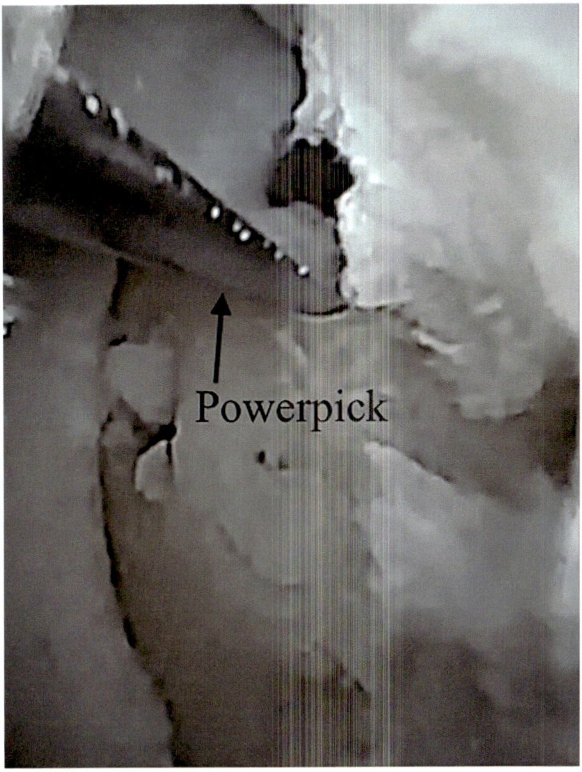

Fig. 2 Viewing the left knee in flexion with the Nanoscope (Arthrex) 0° anterolaterally. You can see the lesion medially and the Powerpick (Arthrex) performing the microfracture

4.4.2 Osteochondral Autograft Harvesting

While viewing from the lateral portal with the Nanoscope (Arthrex) and the knee in full extension a shaver with the GraftNet (Arthrex) applied is placed through the medial portal. It is important to debride as much synovium from the areas of harvesting prior to harvesting to increase the amount of pure cartilage harvested (Figs. 3 and 4). This shaver then is used to harvest the nonarticulating portion of cartilage from the medial femur. The shaver and Nanoscope (Arthrex) are switched and in similar fashion autograft cartilage is harvested from the lateral nonarticulating cartilage of the femur. This autograft cartilage is then removed from the GraftNet (Arthrex) on the back table.

4.4.3 Mixing Composite Graft

1 cc of Biocartilage (Arthrex) is then added to the Biocartilage mixing cannula with the autograft cartilage. 1 cc of bone marrow concentrate is also added and mixed with the graft until a toothpaste consistency is obtained (Figs. 5, 6, and 7). The delivery cannula is then applied to the mixing cannula and this is placed on the back table.

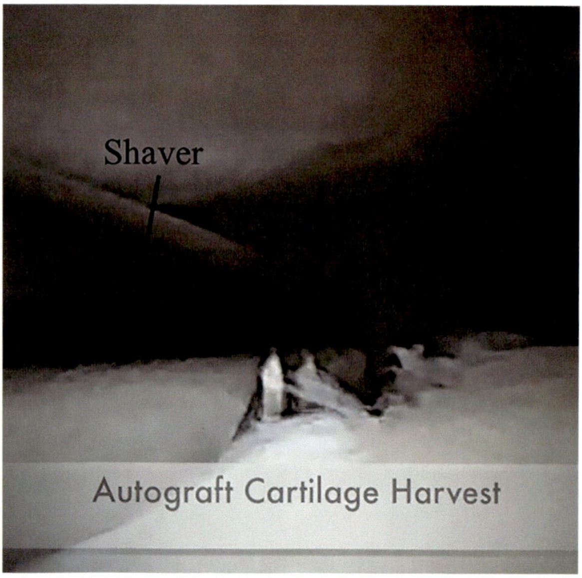

Fig. 3 Viewing the left knee in extension with the Nanoscope (Arthrex) 0° anterolaterally. The shaver with the GraftNet (Arthrex) placed through the medial portal is harvesting autograft cartilage from the nonarticulating cartilage of the medial trochlea

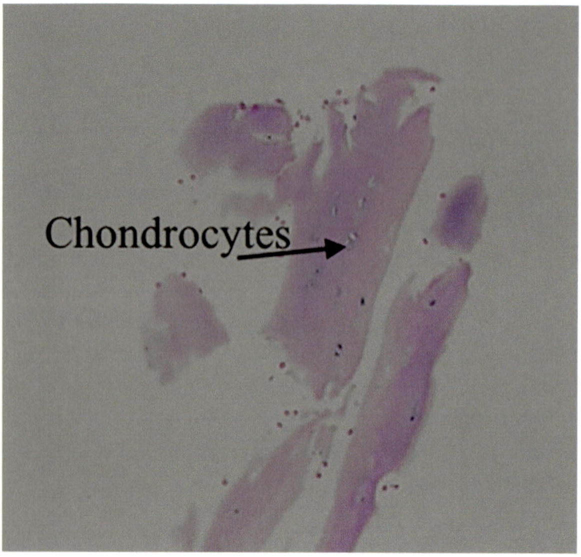

Fig. 4 Histology of the autograft cartilage obtained with hematoxylin and eosin staining at 40x power

4.4.4 Composite Graft Delivery

It may be helpful to establish an inferior accessory portal to aid in suctioning during graft delivery. The arthroscopy fluid is turned off at this point and sponges can be used through the lateral portal to dry the lesion (Fig. 8). The composite graft is then carefully delivered through the lateral portal and a small bone tamp can be used to impact the graft in place. It is important to confirm that the graft

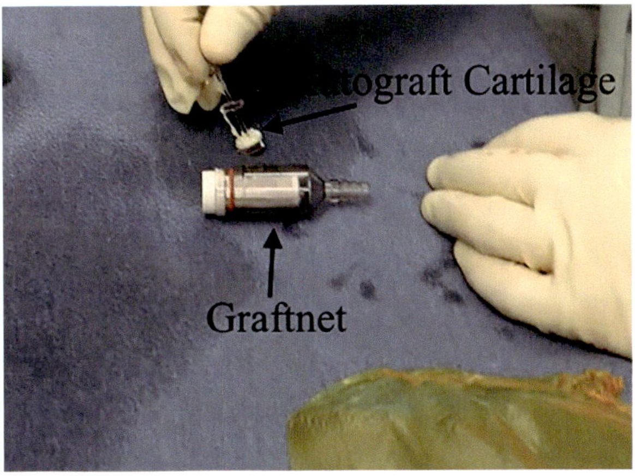

Fig. 5 View showing the autograft obtained and the GraftNet (Arthrex)

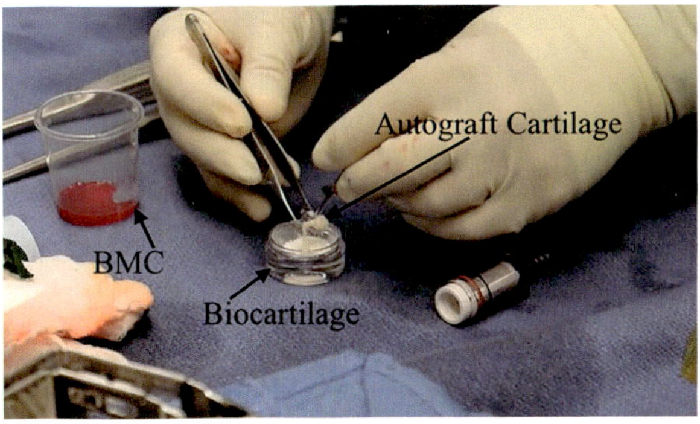

Fig. 6 View from the table showing mixing of the Biocartilage (Arthrex) , BMC bone marrow concentrate, and the autograft cartilage

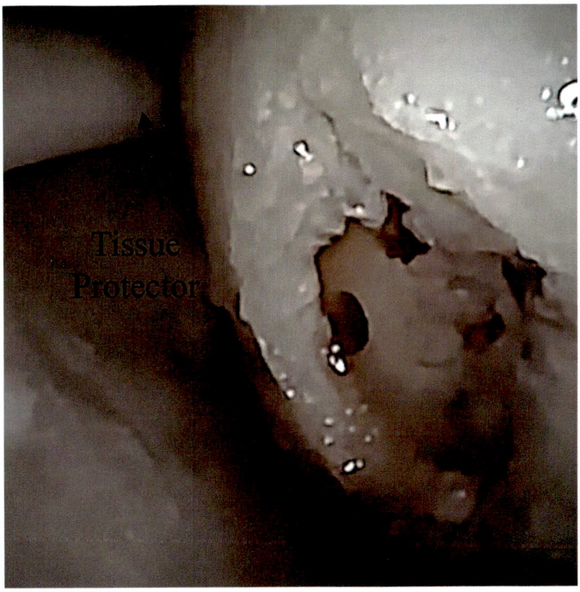

Fig. 7 Viewing the left knee in flexion with the Nanoscope (Arthrex) 0° anterolaterally. You can see the prepared lesion and a tissue protector being used to help keep the lesion dry

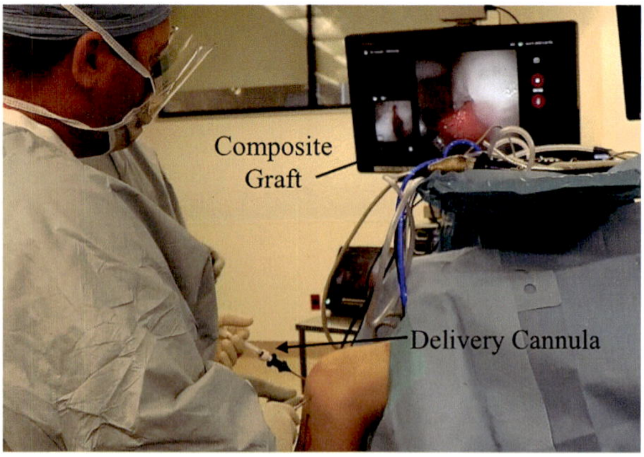

Fig. 8 Viewing from outside the joint. You can see the composite graft being injected on the screen and the delivery cannula is placed into the anteromedial portal

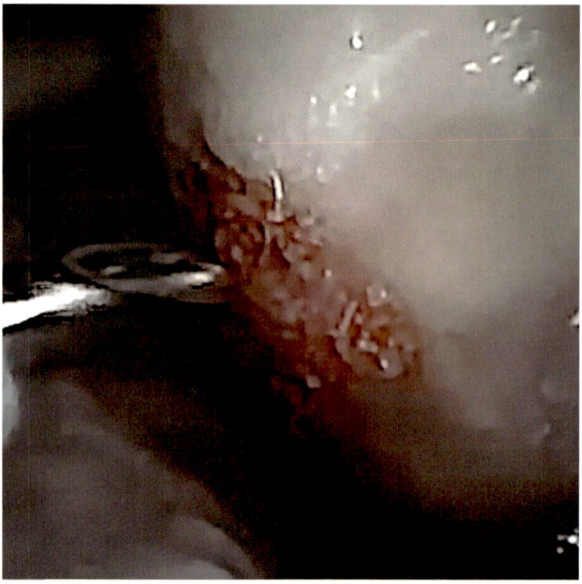

Fig. 9 Viewing the left knee in flexion with the Nanoscope (Arthrex) 0° anterolaterally. The lesion is seen on the medial femur and the Evicel glue (Ethicon) is being delivered onto the lesion

is flush with the cartilage rim and not too prominent on the condyle; this can occur with the delivery of too much graft into the defect. After the graft is properly placed into the lesion Evicel glue (Ethicon, Blue Ash, Ohio) is delivered onto the graft. It is important to start the glue superiorly in the lesion, as it will run inferiorly. (Figs. 9 and 10) Care is taken to not deliver too much glue into the joint; suction can be used to remove excess glue. The glue will need at least 7–8 minutes to set and fix the graft in place.

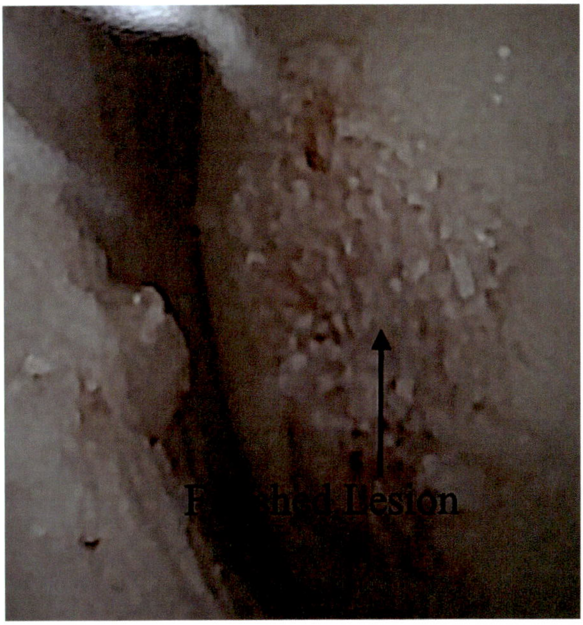

Fig. 10 Viewing the left knee in flexion with the Nanoscope (Arthrex) anterolaterally the final lesion is seen

5 Discussion

Autologous chondrocyte implantation (ACI) aims to restore hyaline cartilage in osteochondral defects without the involvement of subchondral bone. Hyaline content in repaired OCD lesions has been shown to have better outcomes compared to a more fibrocartilaginous fill. Microfracture alone will result in a fibrocartilaginous cap that is able to fill the OCD lesion, but is less similar to the native cartilage compared to the use of autologous chondrocytes with more hyaline concentration. Edwards et al. described the stages and timeline of chondrocyte transfer healing: 0–6 weeks, the implantation phase, has the chondrocytes on subchondral bone protected by the fibrin glue and a large, stable rim. At 6–12 weeks, the transition/proliferation stage sees the chondrocytes migrate into the subchondral bone and begin to fill the defect, forming a primitive repair. From 12 to 26 weeks the chondrocytes undergo remodeling, producing a protein matrix, and becoming a more firm graft. The maturation phase which can last up to 3 years postoperative sees the chondrocytes completely mature with the integration of the graft into the surrounding native cartilage. Recent systematic reviews have shown equal or improved outcomes of ACI compared to traditional microfracture [5, 6]. First-generation ACI was a two-stage procedure where nonarticulating hyaline cartilage is harvested arthroscopically and cultivated in a laboratory, and reimplantation of the matured chondrocytes into the defect during the second-stage operation. Recently, there has been interest in converting this technique into a single-stage procedure by combining harvested chondrocytes with bone marrow concentrate or plasma-rich protein to create composite grafts. This prevents the need for multiple operations and allows decreased donor-site morbidity due to less autograft needing to be harvested. Buda et al. in 2010 reported on 20 patients who underwent single-stage ACI with composite grafting of autologous cartilage, bone marrow-derived stem cells, and platelet-rich fibrin. Two of their patients underwent lesion biopsy and found type II cartilage formation and filling of OCD defect [7]. Cugat et al. in 2017 also reported excellent filling of OCD defects on MRI and arthroscopy in two patients who underwent a similar procedure with the addition of intra-articular PRP injection. Both patients were able to return to their pre-injury level of function [8]. Salzamann et al. in 2017 present a single-stage open ACI technique with cartilage chips and fibrin glue [9]. Our single-stage arthroscopic technique uses the GraftNet (Arthrex) to collect the autologous cartilage in a simple fashion, and combining with BioCartilage (Arthrex) allows for a viable alternative graft without the need for a second procedure [10]. By modifying our previously described technique with the use of the Nanoscope (Arthrex), we can decrease pain and morbidity by using a single incision while still maintaining a working portal for adequate defect preparation and autograft harvest. Another benefit of the Nanoscope is the ease of drying the joint for graft implantation; less flow from the Nanoscope makes a difficult portion of the case easier. Despite the aforementioned benefits the Nanoscope (Arthrex) can be technically demanding. Lesions that are not able to be directly viewed are more difficult to manage. If the lesion is not anterior on the condyle when the knee is flexed it may be difficult to adequately debride and implant the composite graft. Fortunately, the Nanoscope allows for a wider range of visualization angles which can aid in triangulating the instruments to achieve graft placement. Technical pearls include using the high flow sheath, changing the Nanoscope orientation for a better view of a lesion that is not anterior on the condyle, and ensuring that the joint is as dry as possible prior to graft placement. Although studies are needed to assess the long-term results of our technique, we are optimistic that our single-stage, single-incision nanoscopic ACI procedure is a viable procedure that is an improvement over traditional chondrocyte transfer.

6 Editor's View

This chapter represents a technique that is a great combination of the Nanoscope being used percutaneously to view and only making a very small incision to do an autograft cartilage transfer. This is one of the best combination techniques that we have combining the Nanoscope with our updated biologic-type reconstructions utilizing the GraftNet device. Basically, we are taking the autograft cartilage transfer technique which transfers autograft cartilage cells and utilizing the Nanoscope for our viewing portal percutaneously in hopes that this improves patient outcomes. We've had great success with our early outcomes with this approach and look forward to using similar approaches for other reconstructions in the future.

References

1. Detterline AJ, Goldstein LJ, Rue J-P, Bach B. Evaluation and treatment of osteochondritis dissecans lesions of the knee. J Knee Surg. 2008;21:106–15.
2. Grimm NL, Weiss JM, Kessler JI, Aoki SK. Osteochondritis dissecans of the knee. Clin Sports Med. 2014;33:181–8.
3. Engasser W, Christopher LC, Stuart MJ, Krych AJ. Current concepts in the treatment of osteochondral lesions of the knee. Minerva Ortopedica e Traumatologica. 2015;64:459–71.
4. Kocher MS, Tucker R, Ganley TJ, Flynn JM. Management of osteochondritis dissecans of the knee: current concepts review. Am J Sports Med. 2006;34:1181–91.
5. Kraeutler MJ, Belk JW, Purcell JM, McCarty EC. Microfracture versus autologous chondrocyte implantation for articular cartilage lesions in the knee: a systematic review of 5-year outcomes. Am J Sports Med. 2018;46(4):995–9. https://doi.org/10.1177/0363546517701912.
6. Na Y, Shi Y, Liu W, et al. Is implantation of autologous chondrocytes superior to microfracture for articular-cartilage defects of the knee? A systematic review of 5year follow-up data. Int J Surg. 2019;68:56–62. https://doi.org/10.1016/j.ijsu.2019.06.007.
7. Buda R, Vannini F, Cavallo M, Grigolo B, Cenacchi A, Giannini S. Osteochondral lesions of the knee: a new one-step repair technique with bone-marrow-derived cells. J Bone Joint Surg Am. 2010;92(Suppl 2):2–11.
8. Cugat R, Alentorn-Geli E, Steinbacher G, et al. Treatment of knee osteochondral lesions using a novel clot of autologous plasma rich in growth factors mixed with healthy hyaline cartilage chips and intra-articular injection of PRGF. Case Rep Orthop. 2017;2017:8284548.
9. Salzmann GM, Calek AK, Preiss S. Second-generation autologous minced cartilage repair technique. Arthrosc Tech. 2017;6(1):e127–31. Published 2017 Jan 30
10. Lavender C, Sina Adil SA, Singh V, Berdis G. Autograft cartilage transfer augmented with bone marrow concentrate and allograft cartilage extracellular matrix. Arthrosc Tech. 2020;9(2):e199–203. Published 2020 Jan 9. https://doi.org/10.1016/j.eats.2019.09.022.
11. Krill M, Early N, Everhart JS, Flanigan DC. Autologous Chondrocyte Implantation (ACI) for Knee Cartilage Defects: A Review of Indications, Technique, and Outcomes. JBJS Reviews, 2018;6(2):e5. https://doi.org/10.2106/JBJS.RVW.17.00078.

The Future of Nanoarthroscopy

Chad Lavender and Kassandra Flores

1 Introduction

Now that you have been introduced to our newest Nanoscopic techniques in the previous chapters, we can focus on how we take the next step and implement the Nanoscope (Arthrex Inc., Naples, FL) in our everyday practice. This chapter focuses on what is next and what we have learned thus far with the Nanoscope. We will also discuss how I envision an arthroscopy in the future while taking full advantage of the Nanoscope.

2 Diagnostic Nanoarthroscopy

Many surgeons begin Nanoarthroscopy as a diagnostic option. This is one area it shines and makes perfect sense. Because it does not require an incision and should provide a much faster recovery time, when the scope is negative, it works perfectly as a diagnostic device. Some surgeons may decide to use this device in the office to perform diagnostic services. My thought is that we should strive to create environments and techniques that would cut our MRI use in half with the possibility of in-office Nanoscopes. This has several obstacles including billing, sterility, anesthesia, and control of bleeding for visibility. Obviously, the high flow sheath will help with the visibility as we have seen already, but patient selection will be paramount as we travel into the realm of true in-office diagnostic Nanoarthroscopy. What I currently do most in my practice is use it as a diagnostic tool in the outpatient setting. In the immediate future, this is what will help us the most with those difficult to treat

C. Lavender (✉)
Orthopaedic Surgery Sports Medicine, Marshall University, Scott Depot, WV, USA

K. Flores
MS1 Marshall University, Scott Depot, WV, USA

C. Lavender (ed.), *Biologic and Nanoarthroscopic Approaches in Sports Medicine*, https://doi.org/10.1007/978-3-030-71323-2_19

painful joints with negative exams or MRIs. If the scope is negative the patient is immediately cleared without hesitation and if a treatment scope is necessary you can perform reconstructions, repairs, and treatments. So, while we are pushing toward the goal of in-office Nanoarthroscopy, I currently perform the diagnostic exams in operating rooms with anesthesia and do almost 100% of my diagnostic arthroscopies with the Nanoscope.

3 Incisionless or Limited Incision Surgery

As you can see from Part II of the book most of our concentration has been led on creating incisionless or limited incision surgeries. For example with the single incision rotator cuff repair, using the Nanoscope decreased our need for a secondary accessory portal. In addition during the single-incision anterior labrum repair, we were able to do the entire procedure through one small incision. Figure 1 shows Dr. Lavender performing a single incision medial meniscus repair utilizing the Nanoscope. These are major advantages of our standard way of thinking for these types of reconstructions and repairs. In addition to this, performing full incisionless surgeries is now possible. For example, with our partial meniscectomy the patient received no incisions and only spinal needle portals. Our goal moving forward is to continue to stretch the boundaries using smaller implants, smaller devices and to truly live in an incisionless arthroscopy world because of the Nanoscope. Again, with the high flow sheath and our improved flow, which is so vital to Nanoarthroscopy, we are able to perform much larger and more difficult reconstructions where visualization would have previously been much more difficult (Fig. 2). So far this has been where we have really made the most advancement in the Nanoscope and I think we will continue to do so over the next 5–10 years and in the future. In my opinion, the future of Nanoarthroscopy is truly providing patients with fewer incisions, smaller incisions, and therefore improved outcomes.

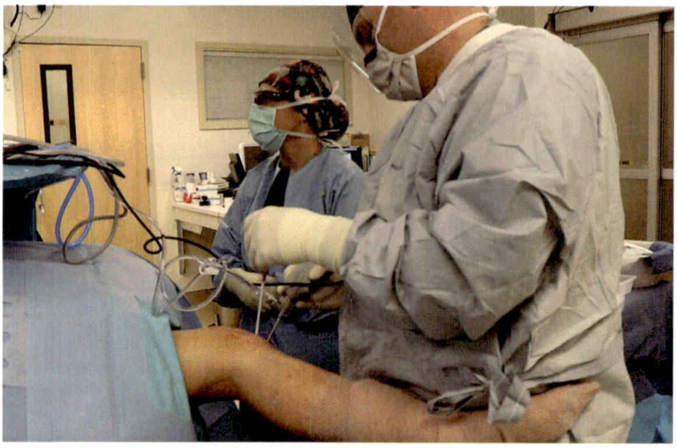

Fig. 1 Dr. Lavender is seen performing a single incision medial meniscus repair utilizing the Nanoscope and the Arthrex Fiberstitch Device. (Arthrex Inc. Naples, FL)

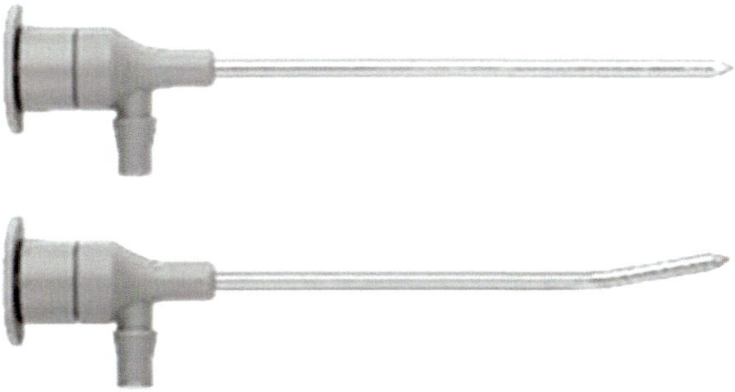

Fig. 2 A view of the high flow sheath and curved high flow sheath available for the Nanoscope

4 Multiple Screen Viewing

Several of our techniques have shown the advantage of using the standard arthroscope as a separate viewing portal to give us multiple visualization fields in the same surgery and multiple viewing angles. I have really worked on when this is necessary, appropriate, and useful and we continue to refine our techniques. This becomes immediately possible if we have several Nanoscopes in various locations throughout the shoulder or knee joint all simultaneously hooked into different screens so that now we can become true 360-degree surgeons at the same time. One correlation could be noted in the video game industry as it went from a two-dimensional to a three-dimensional experience. I see that same correlation with the Nanoscope providing the surgeon with a true three-dimensional view of the joint as they are performing a reconstruction in the future. We can start to imagine multiple screens showing multiple angles of the reconstruction all without the need of portals. This will certainly change the game of arthroscopy and also our outcomes because of the need of fewer portals.

5 Discussion

I think these are the three main areas the Nanoscope will grow in the future and hopefully, as surgeons, we will be excited to grow with the Nanoscope. There will obviously be times that it is not going to be easy to change our viewing habits and surgical techniques, but we have to keep in mind the patient outcomes and the possibilities that lie before us with this great technology. In the second half of this book, we have described several techniques with the Nanoscope, however, that only skims the top of what this Nanoscope is capable of moving forward to in the future as I described in this chapter. This is truly a new frontier in arthroscopy that should be celebrated and embraced for the benefit of our patients.

Index

C. Lavender (ed.), *Biologic and Nanoarthroscopic Approaches in Sports Medicine*, https://doi.org/10.1007/978-3-030-71323-2

Printed by Printforce, the Netherlands